THE INSIDE-OUT MAKEOVER

THE INSIDE-OUT MAKEOVER

✦

TEN TOOLS FOR INNER BALANCE

Andrea Clark, M.A.

iUniverse, Inc.
New York Lincoln Shanghai

THE INSIDE-OUT MAKEOVER
TEN TOOLS FOR INNER BALANCE

iUniverse books may be ordered through booksellers or by contacting:

iUniverse
2021 Pine Lake Road, Suite 100
Lincoln, NE 68512
www.iuniverse.com
1-800-Authors (1-800-288-4677)

ISBN-13: 978-0-595-35738-3 (pbk)
ISBN-13: 978-0-595-80216-6 (ebk)
ISBN-10: 0-595-35738-5 (pbk)
ISBN-10: 0-595-80216-8 (ebk)

Printed in the United States of America

Contents

FOREWORD. vii

INTRODUCTION xi

INSIDE-OUT MEDITATION xvii

TOOLS 1

    A. Counseling 2

    B. Nutrition 10

    C. Acupuncture. 18

    D. Herbal medicine 23

    E. Homeopathy. 26

    F. Chiropractic 30

    G. Exercise 34

    H. Bodywork 40

    I. Breathwork 48

    J. Meditation. 52

CASE STUDIES. 57

    A. Clare: "I don't know what I want" 58

    B. Geoff: "It began with a macrobiotic diet" 61

    C. Miriam: "I do what everyone tells me; why do I still feel lousy?" 64

    D. Barry: "I don't really feel sick; I'm just always tired" 69

    E. Angela: "I've been fat forever; I hate it." 72

RECOMMENDED READING 75

    A. Counseling. 76

    B. Nutrition 78

    C. Acupuncture. 80

    D. Homeopathy 81

    E. Chiropractic 82

    F. Herbal medicine 83

    G. Exercise 84

    H. Bodywork 86

    I. Breathwork 88

    J. Meditation. 89

FOREWORD

When I think back over the decades of my adult life, each seems to have promoted a particular theme. In the fifties, we worked to keep the "status quo"; the seventies were dedicated to the emergence of female power, and good folk music; during the nineties, use of techno-toys emerged. Since the dawn of the new millennium, the makeover has reigned supreme. In this decade of change, anyone with financial resources who posesses relatively good health may alter their environment, wardrobe, hair, teeth, nose or breasts. They may even opt to take themselves to a plastic surgeon who will completely re-sculpt their body.

Usually, we wish to make over our outer environment or our physical body because we hope to alter the way we view our inner selves. Many of us soon discover, however, that revising the cover does not necessarily change the book. After spending thousands of dollars on new furnishings or painful reconstructive surgery, we may still feel inferior, emotionally upset or essentially unchanged. Unfortunately, most TV makeover programs do not depict the misery experienced by those who have sought change, yet still feel that they have not achieved inner perfection. Some continue to subject themselves to surgical alteration, hoping that the next procedure will finally enable them to reach their dream of perfection.

After years of attempts to make ourselves over, we may conclude that the problem with our harsh self-judgment lies not outside us, but deep inside, and that the true makeover will not come from those efforts to improve our external selves. Permanent change can only emanate from within. We all know those people who seem to shine with an inner glow, although they may appear far from perfect on the outside. Their noses may not be straight and narrow; their breasts may be small, or overly large, their weight below or above the ideal. They may live in sub-standard homes, with outdated appliances and furnishings. We wonder how they can possibly be happy, or why their often good-looking spouses adore them.

These people glow because they feel healthy, because they feel content with what they are and have, and because they love themselves for the inner beautiful people they are. They have learned somehow that because they feel beautiful, they are beautiful, and those who are close to them agree. They take in and emit positive experience, nourishing themselves from within and passing on their optimism to others.

When we continue to seek perfection from outside through subjecting ourselves to surgery, acquiring more and more stuff or ingesting pills for weight loss or a diet low in real nutrition, many of us begin to feel toxic. We find ourselves financially wanting, improperly fed, physically dissatisfied, and too often, less healthy than we did when we began our campaign to achieve perfection. And, because our health has been compromised, our capacity for contentment, lightness and joy in our lives is often severely diminished, causing us to feel dis-spirited, or dissatisfied with life.

We usually arrive at this state of dissatisfaction unaware of the reasons we make the choices we do. Why do we fail repeatedly, when we fully intend to succeed? Why do we feel stuck, powerless or out of control? Why do we repeatedly become ill? Why do we feel unbalanced? Where do we turn when our resources are depleted?

When I found myself in the midst of emotional crisis over thirty years ago, many forms of affordable counseling were readily available to help me discover my personal path to self-discovery. Because my insurance plan covered as much therapy as I needed to solve my problems I was able to have regular counseling sessions for over a year. At that time, I was not aware of other tools, probably because many of them were not readily available.

Yoga, bodywork, meditation and acupuncture have become much more popular in the past 20 years. At the same time, counseling has diminished in popularity. This may be due to the expense of regular therapy, or to the fact that this form of healing carries the burden of social stigma. Another reason for the avoidance of counseling is often the use of drugs to alleviate emotional pain. It seems easier for most of us to visit our primary care physician when we need professional help rather than seeking counseling.

Since modern emotion-altering medications do not have the ability to help us unravel certain negative patterns we have deeply ingrained in our psyches, over time these patterns may become deeply, almost cellularly ingrained beliefs. These beliefs may have worked well for those who love and teach us, and we may have adopted them because we put our trust in our teachers.

Those who raise us usually assume we need the social patterns they have adopted in order to cope in this world, as they have. Sometimes, this is true; often, it is not. When the information we have learned does not work for us, and we continue to lead our lives in a manner programmed within us by others, sooner or later we feel out of balance. We then seek help from doctors, who refer us to psychiatrists, who then prescribe complex drugs. After years, dis-eased and discontent with our lives, we feel consistently out of control.

When we reach this stage in our lives, where do we go? Do we opt for more medication, or the acquisition of more things, or more changes to our outer selves? If we do, we soon discover that these paths will not bring us to balance, but in fact may be making us feel worse. What is lacking in these forms of treatment is a way to help us make ourselves over from within in a relatively short time, and without breaking us financially; a way to answer the constant *whys?* in our lives.

We need to learn to become our own inner healers, doing personal detective work to seek the causes of our dis-eases and searching out those tools which are able to aid us in finding our way back to that perfect inner balance which is our natural birthright. Practitioners of the therapies I have included in *The Inside-Out Makeover* hopefully perceive us as complete beings, and are able to work with us to discover the ways in which we keep ourselves unbalanced.

As I traveled my personal path, I discovered that one tool was not enough. Counseling certainly helped me to identify those issues which were causing inner turmoil, but it did not remove them entirely. For years after seeking help for my problems, I found myself frequently returning to negative patterns despite work with excellent therapists, and the ingestion of medication to ease chronic depression and anxiety. At times, I thought I would be in this medication and therapy reliance cycle forever. My mind knew why I was ill, but my body still held on to its dis-ease. I needed to find ways to let go of my illness.

The second tool I discovered was acupuncture, which joined my body, mind and spirit to enable greater balance and healing. A few years later, I found that meditation deepened my ability to relax and focus. Chiropractic work helped to keep my spine aligned and balanced, while bodywork such as massage, reflexology, Reiki and cranio/sacral balancing extended my self-knowledge and hastened physical healing. Recently, I have added herbal medicine to my bag, to root out those toxins which remain deeply embedded within my system.

If we think of the cause of dis-ease as the root of the tree, and the symptoms as branches, why would we wish to continually feed and water only the branches when we could dig deeper to nourish the root? The branches would then naturally heal by drawing on the health of the root. This is the true makeover: discovering the cause of inner dis-ease, and changing it. This change is permanent, and forever.

INTRODUCTION

In the mid-sixties, just after the birth of my son, I was diagnosed with Rheumatoid Arthritis. I was twenty-five. In those days there were two ways to deal with the disease: steroids in the form of Prednisone, and aspirin. I discovered that I was allergic to steroids, so I needed to resort to buffered aspirin. I took 16-20 of these daily, to keep the pain, inflammation and crippling at bay. Because I had a very virulent form of the syndrome, the medication did not slow the crippling. After five years, although I managed to keep pain at a low level, many of my larger joints including my ankles, wrists and neck were fused.

Doctors were amazed at the rapid deterioration of my joints, but could not stop the damage. One rheumatologist told me that I was simply "not the rheumatoid type", and asked if I would appear before a panel of his peers who would discuss my condition. I asked him if he thought they could solve the problem. He told me he did not think so, but they were curious about the development of my condition.

In retrospect, perhaps if I had consented, the investigation into my condition might have helped those who suffered the same fate, but at the time I could not choose to be a lab study for a group of curious doctors who would not guarantee my cure. Instead, I spent a month crying and depressed, then chose to stop seeing doctors, especially Rheumatologists.

I do not recommend that others follow my path, especially since there are medications today which are able to work miracles for those with crippling arthritis. For me, however, it seemed the only solution at that time in my life. I would continue to take buffered aspirin, and would continue with my life, whatever it brought to me. At that time, life seemed to bring a continuing downward spiral. My husband admitted that he was unable to deal with my deteriorating condition, and he did not think he was capable of caring for me and our two small children if I were to become severely disabled. We decided to divorce.

I was aware that I needed counseling to deal with the divorce, so I reluctantly picked up my first tool. A family member who knew I was depressed and anxious about working and raising a family alone recommended a counselor she was seeing, After three months of intense anxiety, I took a deep breath and called her.

My life had become so complicated. Why was I always feeling sick, angry and fearful? I was addicted to multiple substances including tranquilizers, cigarettes, food and alcohol, I suffered panic attacks two to three times weekly, and I alternated between crying myself to sleep and raging at my life.

One of the first questions I was asked by this counselor was, "What do you need from me?" I was overwhelmed. No one had ever asked me that question. That question implied that this person who was sitting in front of me was actually offering to listen to my needs. She did not assume she knew them, or that I might not. We spent the whole first session discussing what that realization meant for me.

The question implied that, number one, I actually *had* needs, and that number two, another person was willing to listen to them, and perhaps to help me to fulfill them. Years later, when I became a therapist, I knew that the first question I would ask my clients would be "What do you need from me?" I found that many of them reacted as I had; they had not heard that question from anyone in their lives.

Other than discovering I could have my needs met, I also learned that I was able to make choices. I could weigh and measure options and choose to say no if I needed to. These two ideas, which until then had been entirely foreign to me, became the underlying structure for my mental health. When we know what we need and state it, and we can say no when we choose to, we feel more personal freedom, and living becomes much more fluid and open.

Armed with my newfound ability to make choices, I decided that there must be alternatives to medicine for my condition. I was still physically disabled, and in pain most of the time. My counselor was seeing an acupuncturist for a chronic physical problem, and shared that following a number of treatments, she felt not only physically but emotionally and mentally better. She suggested I talk with her acupuncturist.

Adopting this tool was more difficult than counseling. My family and friends gave me no support, feeling that I was subjecting myself to "quackery". I knew nothing about the Eastern medical field, and my primary care physician was a relative who did not believe in any type of treatment other than conventional Western care.

Nevertheless, it was my choice, so again I took a deep breath and plunged into the unknown. I talked with the acupuncturist, who was actually not Chinese, but in fact was from Ohio. He recommended reading material to accustom me to this new treatment, and sent me for a thorough evaluation to a Western physician who worked with him. The doctor shared with me that in Eastern terms, I was very "depleted", and although he was worried about my health, he would recommend that I work with Jim, the acupuncturist.

I learned that practitioners of Eastern or holistic medicine view the system as an integrated physical, mental and spiritual whole, and understand the process of disease as a breakdown of the energy, or Chi, of the whole system. They work with the patient to dig deep into the root of the breakdown, and when they discover it together, the patient is able to use herbal medicine, acupuncture or other forms of natural healing to balance the system from the within.

I have also discovered that some practitioners of holistic health may not be true healers. I consider a *true* holistic healer one who firmly believes that whatever healing modality is best for the health of the root, whether it is Eastern or Western medicine, must be investigated. True healers are fully aware that they are never able to know everything about the human system, and are able to admit to their limitations and readily steer clients in whichever direction which may be necessary for their healing.

The true holistic healer often recommends Western medicine. Medication which relieves depression and anxiety while clients accustom themselves to counseling allows more comfort and less stress, and helps immeasurably to begin the person on the road to improved mental health. Western medicines effectively relieve pain, infection, and harmful symptoms of many diseases. When used sparingly, along with alternative deep-healing, a patient can experience a much faster return to robust good health. I also firmly believe that nothing beats scientific medicine when it comes to an emergency situation which requires surgery or other forms of critical care.

Why then do Western medical doctors not work hand in hand with holistic practitioners? Common sense tells me that if they worked together, all of us could conceivably be much more healthy with much less ingestion of medication, not to mention reduced cost to insurance companies and individuals who are treated. There is great merit in both methods of treatment; when I have seen them used together, I have been astounded by the results. I am a product of that use, and the healing I have experienced delights me. I know that one method alone would not have worked for me; I needed the harmonizing melody of Eastern and Western treatment to assure my deeper balance.

When you choose prescribed Western medications on your path to growth, my advice would be to investigate them as fully as you would any other tool you choose to use. Ask your doctor about prevention of long-term side effects, and take medicines wisely, as you would anything you ingest. I have found medications a great help in certain situations. I still use small amounts of two of them on a daily basis. I am aware of the side effects of each, and I protect myself accordingly.

This harmony does exist in some pockets of the country. As an example, there are those physicians like Dr. Andrew Weil, or Dr. Depak Chopra, who employ a combination of treatments to heal and balance. It is my fervent wish that this movement grows to reach all of us as quickly as possible. If you agree with this wish after reading this book, you could become a missionary to good health by sharing your knowledge with your loved ones. Change is difficult for one person, but when there are many in agreement, it occurs much more quickly.

I have continued to discover and add many other tools over the years. It seems that each time I am prepared to journey to a different level, the appropriate tool presents itself to me. After many years, I have come to trust that I do not need to search very far for help; when I need it, it will come to me.

Rabbi Zelman Schachter-Shalomi, in his work with Spiritual Eldering, calls the years after 50 "the third half of life". I am looking forward to ever increasing contentment and ever-improving health during this last half of my life. As part of my personal Spiritual Eldering, I am writing this small book to share the pathways I have found, and have helped others to find, to a greater, more bountiful state of health.

My inner makeover will probably not be yours; you must discover your own. The tools contained in this book will help you to discover your personal path to inner balance. Let me also add that this book is not meant to be ingested page by page. Rather, go to those parts to which you are drawn. Read it a bit at a time if you wish. I do recommend you read the section concerning counseling before you put the book aside, since I consider it a springboard to the tools which may follow.

My aim in writing this book is to provide you with enough information presented in a direct, easy-to-understand format, to start you on a journey to inner balance and self-discovery. Because there are hundreds of treatment modalities available these days, and because I am not personally familiar with many of them, I have chosen to write about the ten "tools" I have directly experienced, with the hope that you will be interested enough to delve deeper into those which appeal to you.

I hope also that the investigation and subsequent use of one or more of these tools will help you deepen your knowledge of your unique self. Remember, each of us is born with the personal tools needed to live life according to our unique destiny. Unfortunately those who raise, love and teach us often do not take our individuality into consideration, and rather than encouraging us to develop into our authentic selves, they often remove pieces of our innate wholeness from us through criticism and false expectation, leaving us feeling empty and unbalanced. We must spend much of our lives regaining that balance.

Each of the tools you utilize is important in itself, but you will probably need more than one to achieve permanent change. There are numerous writings concerning each tool, and many of them would have you believe that if you use one properly, it will work miracles for you. I have taken advantage of all of them, and have realized that while some tools may work quickly and well for me, I felt that others produced little or no change. Since we are all unique, only your personal bag of tools will work for you. I have chosen the specific tools for this book because they have worked well for me, and for those I have been fortunate enough to guide on their paths to wellness.

Please know that although I have not chosen to include certain treatment modalities, it does not mean I do not recommend them. What I do recommend is that if this primer piques your curiosity, take your curious self to the internet, a bookstore or a healing center and delve deeply into research of any and all of those healing treatment methods which may appeal to you.

Since you are already perfect and intact within yourself, the tools provided within are meant to reveal and heal those physical and spiritual wounds which stand in the way of your existing perfection. I am a human being, subject to whatever that means, as are you. For most of us, this means a lifetime of confusion, fence-sitting and feelings of frustration and powerlessness, interspersed with short periods of lightness, joy and contentment. I have become convinced in my short time on this planet that we are meant to feel the joys much more than the frustrations. This is able to happen only if we clear away those blockages in our bodies, minds and spirits which stand in the way of our inner balance, our real selves.

In the first section each tool will be briefly explored, with examples when appropriate. (This is a primer, after all). My hope is that you will more thoroughly investigate those which appeal to you, then place them in your bag to use in your process. Following explorations of the tools, I have presented five case studies, adapted from the many clients I have worked with. Sharing in others' work, knowing you are not alone in yours, often proves a valuable tool. The third section provides a bibliography of readings you may want to use to take your own inner makeover to a deeper level.

A MAKEOVER MEDITATION

Before we begin, since I have derived much benefit from visual therapy, I am providing you with the following inner journey. If you are not familiar with visual imagery, simply read it and notice whether you begin to picture images in your mind. Many people do not see inner pictures, but are able to internalize guided imagery with symbols or words. Know that whatever works for you is entirely correct.

My suggestion is to read the meditation slowly, allowing two or three deep breaths wherever you notice the "pause dots". Return to this meditation any time you feel you need to re-acquaint yourself with the purpose of this book. Good luck on your venture into your self. It could be the most rewarding journey you have ever taken.

JOURNEY TO THE AUTHENTIC SELF

Close your eyes, and begin to pay attention to your breath....Notice, as you listen and become more aware, that your breath deepens and becomes quiet, more steady....you begin to feel more relaxed...concentrate on the sounds you hear outside your body...listen to them, accept them...bring your attention to your outer body, scanning it for any discomfort...now, bring attention to the inner body, relaxing it...you are now very relaxed, and ready for your journey....you are walking slowly down a beautiful, wooded path....this is the path which will take you to ever-increasing contentment and bountiful good health....as you walk along, you see an empty bag of soft, beautiful material in front of you......pick it up and sling it over your shoulder.... This bag is for the tools you will find along the way, tools which will help you to become your true self......further along your path, you begin to see a person walking slowly toward you.... You realize that it is you, but you look different...you glow with health, both outside and in...as the person approaches, notice the differences between yourself and the other...approach each other slowly, and become aware that you are allowing yourself to enter the body of the other......take some time to accustom yourself to this new body...notice that this body feels good to live in....this body is strong, light, well-fed, properly exercised....this body is treated with kindness and appreciated by you....this body loves to touch and be touched.... You also have a healthy mind.......this mind is focused and carries you forward without fear....this mind does not judge, condemn or blame....this mind has creative, constructive, positive thoughts....this mind remains consistently open to new concepts....your spirit is also healthy......this spirit loves and accepts easily...this spirit expresses positive appropriate emotion....this spirit is consistently fluid....this spirit loves to laugh and to play......enjoy this body for a few moments, then step back into the present body...compare your wonderful, healthy body with the body you walk in today......know that you are both bodies....know that whatever you vision, you are....keep this vision with you as you grow....see yourself evolving, becoming more and more the person you are....breathe deeply, and return to your present place.

TOOLS

COUNSELING

At a time when I needed extensive dental work, I traveled to a large inner-city training hospital in Florida, where closely supervised students care for their patients. During one appointment Juan, my personal student dentist, enlisted the help of a lovely young woman who was volunteering at the school, hoping to be accepted as a future dental student. While Juan sought out the supervisor who was consulted after every step in my procedure, we used the time to chat. She asked me what I did for a living. I told her I had been a psychotherapist in New England for many years. "What's that?" she asked.

I was astounded. This intelligent young woman did not know what a psychotherapist was. I told her that probably translated into a Mental Health Counselor. I then asked what she would do if she needed help with a problem in her life. She stated that she had never needed counseling, but she supposed she would see a doctor, and take anti-depressants or some other medication, as some of her friends had.

I realized this must be a panacea for young people in this country; they could simply take a pill, and it would fix everything. If this is a choice, I wondered if they realized that while the new drugs may be amazing in their ability to relieve the symptoms of anxiety and depression, ingesting pills every day for months, even years may not cure a life-long pattern of acting out in a negative manner in specific situations. How do pills keep you from entering abusive relationships time after time? How do they help to improve self-image, after living a lifetime in a critical environment? Short-time relief may be achieved, but the causes for the symptoms may never be addressed.

Many of us may feel discontent, empty, unfulfilled. Consistent feelings of unhappiness and dissatisfaction have been part of life for years. We may lose sleep, be ineffective at our job, cry at odd times, be irritable with those we love. We wake tired in the morning, go to bed weepy at night, and drag ourselves around much of the time between. Our friends become tired of complaints, our partners wish the problem would go away, our children want us to play with them again. Medication has lifted our spirits temporarily, but we continue to sink back into the same black hole after a few months.

Most of the clients I have seen through the years arrived at my office feeling just this way. They came to me for help because there seemed no place else to go. They were usually nervous about meeting with me, and afraid that I might be appalled when I heard their stories, or that I would turn them away because I could not help them. There was often the expectation that I would listen to them and then tell their friends and families just how messed up they really were.

In many cases, the partners or family of those who needed help had expressed disapproval with them because they had decided to see a therapist, and had tried to discourage them with remarks like: "There's nothing wrong with you, you just need to see a doctor"; or, "You're not crazy; why would you pay to see someone?" Or, "I know she or he will tell you it's all my fault, it's always the mother's (or father's or husband's) fault".

Negative opinions regarding counseling can cause you to choose not to ask for help, or to seek help only when there is no other option, rather than talking with a counselor when you first feel that there's a problem in your life which is insoluble, or when you feel you're in a rut, stuck between two choices and unable to move forward. The best time to seek counseling is when you are still able to think and act rationally, rather than waiting until you feel so emotionally crippled that you are non-functional and need someone's help to get you back on your feet as soon as possible.

When would I need counseling? I have found that counseling helps during those situations in which I am not able to make a decision or I feel stuck. I think a great majority of us feel this way from time to time, and if we are lucky we have people in our lives such as clergy or good friends who are able to help us through these minor crises. Unfortunately, many of us feel we can muddle through our minor crises alone, and are likely to wait until we cannot think in a rational manner and do not know where else to turn before we ask for help. Or, we may choose to share our problems with people who mean well, but are not qualified or able to help. If you are fearful of harm from another, or you feel so emotionally unable to cope that you drag yourself to a professional with your head between your knees, ready to end it all, the first person you are likely to seek out is a crisis counselor.

These professionals will see you when you are in dire need, allowing you to emote until you feel more rational and are prepared to share your problems, then they will work with you to quickly formulate a plan to solve your crisis. They are armed with resources such as locations of group meetings for addiction or lists of various medical or legal professionals you may need to assist you. You can often find help for your crisis on telephone hotlines or by calling your local hospital or medical center.

If you feel chronically sad, frustrated and depressed, you may opt for psychotherapy. Psychotherapy is just what it says; therapy for the psyche, or mind. Just as physical therapy or Massage therapy help the body to relax, release blockages to physical health and gain greater range of motion, psychotherapy helps the mind to feel more content, release mental blockages to health, and to experience greater, less fearful range of thought. Physical therapies release, relax and open the body; psychotherapy releases, relaxes and opens the mind.

However, we may easily accept physical therapy, since it works only with the physical body, and does not involve probing the mind. Physical therapy may be uncomfortable, but it will not release personal secrets which have been held in for years. You may experience physical pain, but you will not experience emotional pain. The physical therapist can be trusted not to coerce you to air your dirty linen, as it were. Because of these differences, mental therapy requires a deeper trust between you and the professional. The psychotherapist is not your friend. Rather, they are listeners and problem-solvers, guiding you to discovery of your inner authentic self, that self which is whole, content with life, accepting of all that is unique within you. A psychotherapist rarely offers advice; rather, they supply acceptance of you just as you are, mental pimples and all, and offer guidance to that place where you feel as accepting toward yourself as they do. You enter into a paid contract with a therapist, and as part of that contract everything you say is held in confidentiality. Your secrets are safe with them.

Unfortunately, just as there are those few physical therapists who have caused bodily harm, there are experienced psychotherapists who have betrayed trust or caused mental harm. But the great majority of therapists are well-trained, caring individuals who wish only to help you heal your psychic wounds. Many therapists work in large groups, or are in private supervised practices. Often your therapist is supervised, and may share your case with the supervisor as a group exercise, or privately. This is perfectly legal, and confidentiality is confined to this shared relationship. A therapist is also allowed to share your information with your family or the law, if they feel you will physically harm yourself or another.

You may ask therapists if they share information privately or with a group. If this is not comfortable for you, search for a therapist who practices privately. I also ask that you be aware that if you are reluctant to see a therapist because you may not find the right one, you may never begin to heal. We can always find excuses to keep us safe, to avoid risk. Risk-taking is the most important thing you can do for yourself as you start on your path to wholeness. If you never risk, you never move. Safety guarantees that you stay in your rut.

What types of counseling are available? Many therapists learn to counsel according to their personal preferences. There are those who feel that a client or patient does well with a few intensive sessions geared to immediate problem-solving, while others believe that clients need to commit to longer periods of time in order to effect more permanent change. Some counselors believe in structured therapy, with journaling or homework as part of the process for change. Others employ tools such as creative visualization, relaxation and hypnosis to "speed up" the healing process. Terms for some of these therapeutic modalities include Behavioral, Humanistic, Holistic, Psychosynthesis, Jungian, Rogerian, Freudian. There are also many counselors who train in and utilize several modalities of therapy, which they gear to the needs of each client. Always feel free to ask any professional you work with questions concerning their method of counseling. If you are not comfortable with the explanation or the method, look elsewhere.

How do I know which type is best for me? If you are a natural talker, you may need a person who listens for long periods of time before giving you feedback. If you are shy and reticent, you may opt for an outgoing therapist who will comment on your progress during the session, often asking pertinent questions to urge you on. You may have a particular issue you need to talk through. Short-term goal-oriented therapy is a good choice in this instance. If you need life-altering treatment, long-term counseling may be for you. If you are seeking a therapist who is willing to stay with you until deep-seated life patterns have been permanently altered, you might seek a psychoanalyst, a psychiatrist with a specialty developed by Sigmund Freud which suggests that the client attend two or more sessions weekly for a prolonged period of time.

What qualifications do I look for in a good counselor? I have experienced excellent counseling from many different professionals. Paper qualifications are certainly important, but experience, caring, attentiveness and intuition play enormous roles in good therapy. Often, therapists receive a certain degree because this makes it easier to collect insurance payment for their work. Having a doctoral degree in Counseling Psychology does not always ensure excellent counseling. Psychiatry is actually a specialty following reception of a medical degree which allows the doctor of Psychiatry to prescribe medication. I know a psychiatrist who is an excellent counselor, but this is not always the case. Depending on the state in which therapists choose to work, they may pursue a PhD in Counseling Psychology, a masters degree in social work (MSW), a license in social work (LicSW), a master of arts degree (MA), a master of education degree (MEd), or a training as a mental health worker, which may entitle them to a license (Lic-MHW). Others who counsel are clergy, guidance counselors in educational facilities and those who are trained to work on hotlines. Last but often not least, there are always those we love and trust, our friends and families.

The most valuable quality of any good therapist is their ability to be present with you. This means that you feel that your counselor is totally aware of you and your issues. They listen intently and give you appropriate feedback, and you feel completely at ease, cared for and most important, *heard*. Often clients seek out a therapist because they feel no one really pays attention to them. Attention does not mean the professional simply stares at them quietly; it means that they attend to each client's needs in whatever way the client needs them. You will be aware when a counselor is not there; you may feel you are simply wasting their time, or perhaps they are ready for the session to end, or you may need to repeat something two or three times. If you are not attended to, your therapy will not be as effective. You have the right to end the therapy if you feel this way.

How much will counseling cost? I ask my clients to think of their time in therapy as an investment in their mental health. I often compare an investment in therapy to the purchase of a major appliance, for example a refrigerator. A good refrigerator can cost over a thousand dollars. Most of us pay for it on time, a certain amount of dollars monthly. When we do this we actually pay more than the price of the appliance, since we also pay interest. And, no matter how good it is, after 10 to 15 years, it will need replacement. Good psychotherapy costs money, either weekly or monthly, but there are no interest charges. And, after 10 to 15 years, having gained the tools to change your life, you continue to improve. You may want to work out an affordable payment plan in advance with your therapist. Many counselors will accept insurance plans if yours covers therapy, and if they do not, they may agree to accept payments after you have completed your counseling contract with them. Or they may work with a sliding fee scale, allowing you to pay what you feel you can afford. Please note that although psychoanalysis is very helpful in many cases, it can pose a financial burden due to the time and number of sessions involved.

How long will it take? Crisis counseling usually lasts between one and three sessions. Short-term counseling can take anywhere from 6 weeks to 6 months. Long-term counseling can last from 6 months to 3-4 years. Psychoanalysis can take a lifetime. I have known patients who have been in psychoanalysis for over 15 years. Many of us who have sought help often begin with crisis counseling, and later seek a counselor who will help us to make more permanent changes in our lives. Following intensive counseling, you may want to return for a session when you feel it necessary. Check with the counselor to make sure they have a policy of return, since some counselors feel that when therapy for a particular issue is ended, they need to terminate their professional relationship with the client, and feel it best that you do not plan to return for further therapy with them. If you need further counseling, you will need to find another counselor. Counselors may also choose to terminate treatment if they feel you need an opposite sex counselor, if you both agree that you are not improving, if there are issues of non-compatibility or if they move or change their practice.

How do I locate a counselor? Looking for the right therapist is like shopping for a good shoe. You can pay a lot for shoes, but if they don't fit just right, you won't benefit from them or wear them. Word of mouth can be the best way to locate a good therapist. If you are comfortable with this, ask your friends and co-workers who they might recommend. If not, ask your physician or clergyperson, or call a local hotline or medical center. When a person is satisfied with service they have received they will tell others about it. Once you have located a professional, ask if they offer a free interview. This is a good way to find out if you are comfortable with the therapist. If you feel nervous or frustrated after your meeting, I recommend that you look elsewhere. If this therapist does not ease your mind within a half hour, you will probably not feel comfortable working with them long-term.

Long-term therapy involves a strong personal relationship based on deep trust. If you decide to work with a therapist, and feel "pushed" or "rushed" after a few sessions, or you begin missing appointments, you might reconsider working with them. Change is very difficult, and each of us changes according to our unique timing. Some therapists may have the expectation that you are not changing according to their timing. The therapist's personal ego needs are then interfering with your therapy, and you will both experience frustration in a short time. Believe me, there is relief on both sides when this is true, and therapy is terminated. A comfortable fit is necessary for both you and your therapist, so there are times when a professional will inform a client that working together may not be the best path for either of them. If you hear this, be grateful that the therapist was honest with you, rather than allowing you to spend precious growth time and money in vain.

What about group therapy?. Group therapy means exactly what it says. People meet, usually weekly, with a qualified leader. Groups may be formed to resolve a single issue, such as eating disorder or addiction, or to discuss each member's separate issues in a supportive environment. The size of the group usually depends on the leader's preference. A group may consist of five to fifteen members. The positive aspects of group therapy include support of many people and reduction in cost for weekly therapy. The down side of therapy in groups is that some are reluctant to share their issues with a group of people, since confidentiality may be a problem. Also, there may not be enough time in a large group for each person to work on issue resolution. If group therapy appeals to you, check with local mental health centers for information.

What is coaching? Many people are turning to coaching as a form of counseling. We are familiar with one famous coach, Dr. Phillip McGraw. Others who coach the general public include Dear Abby or Carolyn Hax, well-known advice columnists. Coaching is counseling which employs large doses of advice. Dr. Phil parades people with problems who are willing to reveal them in a public format before us, or he may use the media to teach those who watch him as a group. Dear Abby publishes letters from her readers in which they outline their personal problems. Those who write "how-to" books often provide a form of coaching. Private coaches accomplish essentially the same thing with one client at a time, or in small groups. Costs for private coaching are comparable with those of psychotherapy.

The positive aspects of public coaching include free access to a qualified professional who is able to supply you with tools needed to change negative patterns, and also exposure to "clients" who share your problems, with the result that you often discover your issues are shared with many others. The downside of Coaching is that it often does not take into consideration each "client's" unique makeup, and that it also does not always supply enough tools to ensure deeper balance. So, although you may succeed for a short time when you follow a public or private coach's advice, you may find yourself sliding back into negative patterns within a few months.

I am always pleased when I hear Dr. Phil offer to supply "follow up" services for a participant, since I am often aware that the person may not experience permanent change unless he seeks further therapy. Programs like Dr. Phil's have received criticism, but I am gratified to see some form of counseling being offered to the public. Millions of people receiving well-considered, free advice whether it be from television or the newspapers has to be a good thing. If it accomplishes nothing else, it will supply an awareness which you did not possess before you watched or read the coach's advice to his "client".

Once you have located a counselor you are comfortable with, your path to inner balance becomes wider and more open. You are now on your way, with your first tool tucked into your bag. I wish you continued good luck on your inner journey!

NUTRITION

When I began this writing, I preferred to name this tool "good food" but when I thought it over, I realized some might think I was writing about food which tastes good. I am, in some sense, but my goal in presenting this tool is to share my philosophy concerning food in general. I have studied with and read the works of many excellent nutritionists, and I have come to realize that for the most part they have adopted a philosophy that works for them. I have discovered that most of us do this. What works for us, we feel, is sure to work for everyone. I am fairly certain that they all mean well, and wish to help others, but unfortunately, when we decide to follow another's path, it usually does not work for us. We adopt diet after diet, read book after book; all state that they really have the answer for us. And because we are human, after all, and would love to have someone else solve our problems for us, we want to believe that this is so. Finally, someone has done it, and our lives will be changed forever when we follow these directions.

For some, this approach works. These are the lucky ones. Their inner needs match the philosophy set down by another, and their lives are instantly improved. But for most of us, it is just another dead end on the path to self-improvement. We discard a book or diet which does not work, and look for another. Hopefully our search is satisfied in time.

I have discovered that the search becomes much less difficult if you take time to know yourself before you begin it. When you peel off the layers of non-you, and the authentic core begins to emerge, you become more knowledgeable concerning your real wants and needs. The you who is constantly searching may pick up one book, while the authentic you already knows that this will not help in your search for deeper balance. As you continue to develop, your personal philosophy, that one which suits you exactly, will present itself to you.

The field of nutrition is highly documented with facts which often contradict each other. One concept for feeding yourself says that you need to ingest lots of protein and fat, and disregard carbohydrates. Another says that you need a certain balance percentage of carbohydrates, fats and proteins; another says you must not eat any more than a very small percentage of fats. There are those who state that meat and animal products are damaging to our bodies, and those who state that we absolutely need them to survive and be healthy. Many of you have adopted one or more of these philosophies, and have experienced severe digestive, organic or elimination problems after following them for a number of months.

There is also the difference between the Western and the Eastern diet to consider. Western philosophy states that all bodies are able to follow one well-balanced diet and maintain vigorous health; Eastern nutrition states that each body is very different, and that even if two people suffer the same symptoms of disease, they will not necessarily benefit from the same diet.

Traditional Chinese Medicine physicians develop diets for their patients based on their individual energy systems. These diets are based on factors such as the innate temperature of foods, which range from cold to level to hot. The Chinese believe that all foods need to reach a temperature of 100d. in the stomach to digest well. When foods are too cold, or too hot, the stomach needs to work very hard to break them up, and digestion breaks down as the person ages. Complex grains, vegetables and very small amounts of dairy, fish and meat keep the stomach and spleen working efficiently. Sugar, large amounts of red meat, iced drinks, processed foods such as white flour and too much dairy food break down the digestive process. No wonder the Chinese feel that the Eastern spleen/stomach system is often very unhealthy!

I feel that good eating is essential to good health. I also believe that a food plan which works well for *me* often will not help *you*. Realizing this, I will attempt to stay away from your needs and to share the process which brought me to the realization of my needs. I have listed many good readings in the Resources section in the back of the book. My suggestion is that you spend some time in a large bookstore; get a cup of tea, preferably green, and leaf through some of them, or access a couple of pages on the internet. If one appeals deeply to you, go for it. If you are still at sea, keep searching out your authentic self until you discover your path to the best nutrition plan for you.

What is food? Food is the substance we all need to stay alive. That is why those diets which often severely limit food intake are so difficult. If you decide to give up cigarettes or alcohol, you are able stay completely away from them. You cannot avoid food. Those who try often become obsessive anorexics, and a certain percentage of them die of starvation. Aside from being necessary for life, food is often a supplier of positive emotion, a substitute for negative emotion, a social necessity, a path to poor health, a path to excellent health, and/or a delightful treat for the palette.

Food includes anything ingested by mouth which contains nutritional value. Therefore, herbs and vitamin/mineral supplements are also foods. The function of supplements is exactly what the name implies; they supplement our regular diet. That's why it is best to ingest them at mealtimes. The problem with the food most of us take in is that its value is severely depleted, so although it may taste wonderful, it is often not supplying us with proper nourishment.

Many health providers believe there is no need to supplement our diet with extra vitamins and minerals. They are convinced that we get all of the nutrients we need in our diet. This would certainly be true if we were able to ingest a perfectly balanced diet consisting of fresh, pure, unprocessed, unadulterated foods. Many nutritionists believe that we need to eat only these pure, organically grown foods to be truly healthy. I have worked to improve my health for over thirty years, and my philosophy lies somewhere between these two belief systems. I will outline what works for me, what I recommend to clients, and you may judge for yourself which path to choose.

What liquids are best? Water is the best liquid you can take into your system. That said, make sure your water is filtered, and free of extra chlorine and chemicals. For years I believed we need lots of water daily, but recently I have changed my convictions, after learning through Eastern practitioners that the kidneys and the system in general function better when we "drink to thirst", which means ingesting water at room temperature when we feel thirsty. Drink slowly and stop when thirst is satisfied.

Whole fruit and vegetable juices are fine in small quantities, but they need to be mixed with water to cut down on their high sugar or nutritive content. If you tolerate caffeine, green tea is a good choice, since it is loaded with anti-oxidants, those substances which help move ingested substance through the body quickly and efficiently, so that foods which are not so pure are not allowed to stand and stagnate, causing problems down the line. If you love and tolerate coffee, remember that caffeine is a drug, and too much of it may become addictive. One or two cups of organic coffee daily will probably be well tolerated by a healthy system

What are processed foods? Processed foods are those which have lost much or all of their nutritional value because vitamins, minerals and other micro-nutrients have been removed from them, and in many cases replaced with synthetic products. One of the main reasons for the processing of food is to give it a longer shelf life. Another is to make it look or taste better, so it will beckon to the consumer. Often artificial coloring or flavoring, hardened fats or extra salt or sugar are added to these foods to increase their taste and eye appeal.

Over-processed, depleted food is never good food. The Chinese call this "wrecked" food. Our eyes and taste buds love it, but our bodies do not. We may choose it mostly because we are unable to resist it, but the more whole, unprocessed food we ingest, the more healthy we feel. This includes whole grain breads and cereals, fresh or fresh-frozen vegetables and fruits, organic eggs, free-range poultry, organic dairy products, snacks made with whole ingredients.

Beef and pig are not healthy meats in this country as a rule. They are often injected with massive doses of antibiotics and hormones to keep them from disease and make them bigger and fatter. These substances may affect our health. Lamb can be a good choice, if you can find a supplier who breeds free-range sheep. Buy butter and use small bits of it, rather than processed spreads. Use real maple syrup on your pancakes, but use it sparingly.

One of the most addictive foods available is high-fructose corn syrup. Eating this in large quantities may cause heightened sensitivity to all sugars. Be aware also that sugar is sugar, whether in the form of honey, maple syrup, concentrated fruit juice or refined white sweetener. Ingesting too much sugar causes the pancreas to overwork, putting out insulin to regulate the blood. When the pancreas has worked too hard for too long, insulin production becomes depleted, wreaking havoc with the blood sugar and causing type 2 diabetes.

While it is good for us to consider putting whole foods into our systems, we also need to take the Western lifestyle into consideration. Many of us lead rushed lives, and are unwilling or unable to take the time to purchase and prepare completely balanced meals. And although many supermarkets are expanding their organic food sections, most do not stock large amounts of pure foods, and when they do they can be prohibitively expensive. So we are, in fact, stuck with the foods supplied to us. The most we can do is to make sure that we buy those foods which will harm us least.

My suggestion is to avoid foods with trans-fats (those which are hardened, partially hardened or hydrogenated), foods which list sugar as one of the first four ingredients or contain high-fructose corn syrup, grains from which the nutrients have been stripped and synthetically replaced, meats with large amounts of additives to enhance color and taste and irradiated foods of all kinds. Buy foods in the organic section of the market, and request more accessibility to organic produce and foods.

This does not mean that you need to throw out everything in your pantry and freezer. Remember the mantra: change is difficult. I caution my clients to begin slowly, substituting one food at a time. Eat any food you love once in a while. For example, many people love beef. My husband is one of them. Although I rarely serve it at home, he opts to eat a large hunk of prime rib at a good restaurant once or twice a year. He loves every bite, and it does not disagree with him. I find that for me the trouble with being a "purist" or eating a diet which consists completely of unprocessed organic food (I tried it for a short time) was that cravings took over after a while, and I ended up binging on a food I could not go without for one more day (like pizza).

How do I choose supplements?. There are thousands of supplemental products on the market. You can buy them at your local health food store, on the internet, or through mail-order companies. There are no government regulations on most vitamin or mineral supplements. I agree with the lack of regulation, since regulation may involve an inordinate amount of political intervention. These are foods, after all. But just as some whole foods do not agree with us, there are many food supplements which may cause unwanted reactions.

For example, just because a nutritionist or diet expert states that large doses of vitamin C are best for us does not mean they are. Just because many people you know are taking a certain herb to help memory does not mean that it will help your memory. Be aware that if you are taking any medicinal substance which is meant to thin the blood, and you add herbs like bilberry or ginko biloba, the herbs are likely to exacerbate the effects of the blood thinner. Other substances which can cause the blood to thin are vitamin C, vitamin E and some anti-oxidants. Ginger is often recommended to aid digestion, but if you suffer from heat in your joints or other parts of your body, ginger can add to your discomfort since it is a hot food, and exacerbates inner heat. I speak further about this in the Acupuncture and Herbal tool sections.

Supplements are a wonderful addition to your regular diet, when used correctly. The best way to know which supplements are right for you is to consult a nutritional counselor. Those who are able to help you to develop a good program using supplements include doctors of Chiropractic, qualified nutritionists who work in health food stores, herbalists, doctors of Traditional Chinese Medicine, naturopathic physicians and acupuncture practitioners.

I do not recommend planning a program after merely reading a book on nutrition, since the information in the book, no matter how professional and well thought out, will not take your unique makeup into consideration. Unlike animals, we are not meant to ingest the same diet as others, even those in our own families. My husband and I have diametrically opposite tastes and needs for certain foods. We need to consider this when we eat together at home, and make adjustments as needed, or one of us is likely to eat a totally unbalanced diet.

What method of eating works for you? Since I promised not to recommend a particular food regimen, I will instead share my favorite way to eat. And since this involves ideas taken from a method of feeding yourself which has recently appeared on the bookshelves, I will mention it briefly. (Remember, this has worked for me, and may not work at all for you). I recently read about a new "diet" (one, like a fool, is born every minute). This one is called The Joy Diet. The two major rules of this eating program are: A. Love what you eat, and B. Eat what you love. I had not read the book, and a friend and I shared a chuckle over the premise one day after reading a short article about it. Later, I realized that the idea behind it made sense to me. The philosophy behind this program closely matches the way I have chosen to feed myself after eliminating what seemed like thousands of programs which did not work.

For example, I usually choose to eat pizza as a rare treat, because I have found that both spicy tomato sauce and cheese do not always agree with me, and I work to avoid white bread, since it contains so little usable nutrition. Right there are three foods I feel my body does not need. I am, however, not willing to give up pizza entirely, since I truly love it, so I probably choose to eat it two or three times a year. I realized when I pondered it that if I eat pizza that rarely, it does not disagree with me. In fact, I enjoy every bite of it, because I love it. I also realized that when I used to eat pizza at least once a week, I thought I loved it, but my body certainly told me it did not. I would usually suffer acute indigestion and arthritic pangs for a couple of days following pizza intake. *So, if I truly love what I eat, it means that my body must love it also, since it is not separate from my mind.*

I realized that the two rules Martha Beck uses in her book are the basis of my philosophy concerning the ingestion of food. You need to discover those foods your body/mind truly loves to make you happy, then choose these foods when your body/mind truly wants or needs them. The body/mind is then eating a joyful, health-oriented diet.

For me, loving what you eat and eating what you love means you educate your body/mind to put into it those foods which don't just beckon to you with their smells and look, but which nourish you both physically and emotionally. How many times have you wanted a certain food, then when you eat it feel satisfied after a few bites? You finish it, because you paid for it, or because you took time to prepare it. Don't. Eat only what you really love, while you still love it, then quit. You are training your will to build a more healthy attitude toward food, and your body to tell you when enough is enough. If you feel dissatisfied following a meal and look for more food later, you may not be eating foods you love. Loved foods usually leave us totally satisfied, even when we do not finish them.

This philosophy may not work for everyone. There are some of us who have severe food allergies or chronic illnesses, and need to avoid even those foods you love. Or we have eaten a non-nutritive diet for so many years that substances like sugar trigger a need to eat that won't quit, and we need to stay away from sugar in order to control our food intake. These are severe food imbalance problems, and I have found that many of them subside as the system becomes more balanced overall. If you fall into these categories, you are still able to practice the rules. Within those foods you tolerate, choose those you love most, and eat until the love is fulfilled. Prepare good foods well, chew and digest them slowly and with relish, and cease when your body has had enough.

Following the plan outlined above, I am much more happy with the food I eat. I love what I eat, and eat what I love, about 70 per cent of the time. The rest? Well, I am human, and I am not a purist. I am involved in a constant balancing process, and if I am unbalanced for a short time, my job is to find my way back.

What are "beckon" foods? As part of my education toward a degree in nutrition, I joined a group of women with eating disorders in the Boston area. At one meeting, the leader taught us about "beckoning" food. Beckoning food is that which we have not considered eating until we see it or hear about it. For example: it may be close to lunchtime, and you are considering having a bottle of water and a salad made with lots of greens and veggies and perhaps some grilled chicken added for lean protein. You walk by a bakery on the way to the salad place, and spy a large piece of coconut-frosted chocolate cake in the window. Any thought of salad breezes out of your mind, replaced by the need to eat that cake. You give in to the need, eat the cake as your lunch. The cake actually tastes rather bland but contains three times the calories in the forgotten salad. Three hours later you yearn for a meal of good solid, nourishing food. It's now mid-afternoon, and you have no time to go out. You grab a handful of candy from that dish which always sits full in the break room, washing it down with a cup of vanilla-infused espresso, which you cannot refuse because it smells so darned good. By the time you get home from work, you are so hungry you grab the first food you see, a stale half-bagel on the countertop, lather peanut butter on it and wolf it down to ease your empty feelings and your jagged nerves.

This is beckon eating. It has nothing to do with the joy of eating what you love and loving what you eat. Perhaps you do not really love the thought of the salad, either, but choose it because you need to lose a few pounds, and it seems a healthy option. Perhaps what you would really love for lunch is a pannini sandwich with grilled chicken and roasted veggies. I suggest you eat this if it is what you love. Chew each bite, tasting it fully. Eat as much of it as your body/mind really desires. This may mean half of the sandwich, since the second half begins to fill you to the point where you feel a little uncomfortable. Your body then does not love it any longer. Take the second half home and feed it to your dog, who will fully appreciate it. Or, learn to leave it.

How do I choose a weight-loss diet? I have one word concerning dieting for weight loss; ***DON'T.*** Most diets are unbalanced, and others may not fit your unique needs. If you are having a problem with your weight, see a nutritional counselor and plan an exercise program tailored especially for you. Commit yourself to a lifetime of healthy eating and deeper balance, and your weight will stabilize to suit your body needs. When clients ask me to recommend a diet, I half-jokingly tell them the only diet I support is the ELMM diet. Eat Less, Move More. Severe obesity is an unbalanced condition, but so is a thin condition which does not feel right to your body/mind. Walk that path to your authentic self, which will include the shape and size you are meant to live with.

ACUPUNCTURE

The method of acupuncture known as "Five-Element" was the second tool I placed into my bag. Acupuncture was recommended to me by a counselor I was seeing over twenty-five years ago. She was aware of my physical problems as well as my issues with chronic anxiety, depression and panic attacks. I had gained much awareness of my psychological patterns while we worked, but the physical and emotional symptoms persisted. I decided to try this foreign form of treatment, since western allopathic medications were not helping me get to the source of my illness.

Following a complete evaluation of my energy, Jim McCormick, the acupuncturist recommended I see a physician who was able to understand my energy as he did, by "taking my pulses". Jim did not feel he wanted to begin treatment until I had been seen by someone who could assure him that I would not die while in his care. That doctor informed me that my liver and kidney energy was very low, and asked me what I planned to do if I was not able to take Acupuncture. I shared with him that I felt I had no where to turn, since I did not wish to ingest more medication, and I had no other way of healing. He recommended treatment with the provision that he supervise Jim to make sure I was not getting worse.

Although I was very scared, I also felt deep inside that I was doing something positive for myself. I received three treatments a week for three months, then one treatment a week for the next six months. Fortunately, treatments then were very inexpensive, and Jim worked from his home, so he was able to give me a further break. After nine months of continual treatment, I began to feel very different. I remember sitting in Jim's waiting room one rainy fall morning, thinking about the future. I imagined many roads opening before me, and I was not afraid to take one of these roads to change. To me, since I had lived in fear for many years, this vision felt like an epiphany.

What was actually taking place was a gradual change in inner balance. Because my energy was running more smoothly through my system, it was allowing the healing of inner functions, mainly my digestive, elimination and circulatory systems. I had learned that each of these systems is connected to a major emotion. The liver/gallbladder energy is connected to anger; the kidney/bladder system is connected with anxiety and fear; the circulatory system is connected to contentment and joy. When these systems are working smoothly, emotions become more manageable.

I was able to stop taking prescribed tranquillizers just over a year after I began treatment. I stopped experiencing migraine headaches just after my sixth month of treatment, and bladder and yeast infections ceased after 9 months. I continued to take medication for the joint and muscle pain of rheumatoid arthritis, but the structural damage that was destroying my large joints slowed considerably within two years.

Presently, I receive acupuncture 6-8 times a year, to maintain inner balance. A few years ago, I took a workshop in Boston conducted by SOPHIA, the School of Five Element Acupuncture in Maryland, at which Jim led a few of the exercises. I told him at that point that I was sure he had saved my life. If he had not taken a chance with me so many years ago, I am certain that I would not be here now. He chuckled and assured me that my quality of life was as much my responsibility as it was that of any practitioner, and he would not take credit for my life.

What is acupuncture? This practice of inserting thin needles just under the skin to change the system's energy flow began in China over 3000 years ago, and is used throughout the world as a proven method of discovering the cause of— and in many cases curing— disease, and maintaining healthful balance.

Acupuncturists diagnose problems by placing their fingers gently on multiple pulses in both wrists and lower arms, and "read" the energy in each organ system through the messages these pulses convey. While most of us are able to take, or read, only one pulse in our wrist, Acupuncturists learn to diagnose using other, more subtle pulses. These pulses are indicators of energy "lines" called meridians which run through the body. There are fourteen basic meridians. Twelve of them are connected to our organ energy and two to energy which runs up our spine and down our frontal torso. When the pulses are normal for all of our meridians our bodies are robustly healthy. Unfortunately one or more of our pulses are usually not operating perfectly; this causes systemic imbalance. Perfect body balance is very difficult to achieve, and even more difficult to maintain. We would need to be perfect humans to have perfect pulses all of the time; this is usually not the case.

When acupuncturists discover imbalance, they then determine whether the energy in the meridian is excess, called *yang*, or depleted, called *yin*. They may also determine other factors concerning energy, such as whether it is rising or sinking, hot or cold. When diagnosis is completed, they will choose "points", or places along the lines of the meridians, into which they will insert needles. The needles may be inserted and removed quickly or left in for a time. Depending on the acupuncture method employed, they may use only 4 to 8 needles, or many more. I have experienced treatment using more than 20 needles.

Wherever needles are inserted, energy will be re-directed. Stagnant energy which is not moving will begin to move, and energy which is moving too fast will begin to slow. The entire system will gradually respond, since it has an innate need to become balanced.

Will the needles hurt? Most acupuncture needles are hair-thin, and all are completely safe. Each needle comes sanitized and wrapped, and the practitioner quickly unwraps each needle and inserts it without touching the point.

Since we are all unique, we have unique reactions to needling. In some forms of Acupuncture there is no feeling when needles are inserted, although you may feel warm, or cool, or your extremities may tingle while the needle is in place, or after it has been removed. In other forms you may feel a definite prick when the needle is inserted, since the practitioner is placing it directly into the point. On rare occasions, insertion of a needle will draw a drop of blood, or there may be a small bruise at the site. In over twenty-five years this has not happened to me more than ten times.

When I began to receive acupuncture I was afraid of needles. I found if I lay back, closed my eyes and did not watch the insertion process, I was hardly aware of a needle piercing my skin.

What types of acupuncture are there? Many treatment philosophies have emerged through the centuries. China, Japan and Korea all have highly developed modalities. Needling and reading of pulses are almost universally used, but each method may use other ways of re-directing energy as well. Many Acupuncturists use moxa, an herb which is applied to the skin and heated just before needling to deepen the effect of the treatment. Others use slight electronic jolts to stimulate energy. There is a Japanese treatment which has virtually eliminated use of needles, using only the inner energy of the practitioner and the patient to direct healing into the meridians through the points. The practitioner will usually place either a finger or a needle on the acupuncture point, removing it when the energy is balanced Combinations of modalities have been effectively adapted and passed on by creative modern teachers and practitioners.

I have experienced four types of acupuncture: Traditional Chinese, Korean, Five-Element and Japanese. The philosophy of Chinese Acupuncture is to balance the organ systems, which then leads to balance of the entire structure. Five-Element and Korean Acupuncture approach balance by assuming that the entire structure is composed of the energy influence of five major elements, which constantly interact with each other. These elements are wood, fire, earth, metal and water.

Practitioners usually use one system, but you may find an Acupuncturist who has decided that a combination of two or more treatment modalities seem to heal on a more complex level. I am fortunate to work with two Acupuncturists who use a combination of traditional Chinese, Five Element and Japanese treatment. The combination works very well for my energy. Know, however, that each method is extremely effective, and when you decide to commit to treatment with any modality it will lead to deeper inner balance.

What is acupressure? Acupressure is a means of changing energy in the meridians by exerting pressure on the points with the fingers or other blunt tools, either by pressing deeply or rubbing the points. Since needles are not employed, those who have fear of needles may choose this method of balancing the body's energy.

Acupressure is good for symptom relief, and it may be self-applied. To achieve results, the points may need to by held or rubbed for a period of time two to five times daily. Both acupuncture and acupressure change the energy in the entire system by stimulating the flow at point sites, but because needles are inserted in points rather than the point sites being pressed or rubbed, results are often deeper and faster with acupuncture treatment.

Acupressure may be very effective when used properly, and is fairly easy to learn. There are a number of well-written books which teach you how to treat yourself for many symptoms. Symptomatic relief is fairly easy to achieve with acupressure, but this treatment may not be deep enough to allow the patient to experience permanent balance of the whole system, or recover from long-term chronic illness.

How do I choose an acupuncturist? A master of acupuncture attends an accredited college of Acupuncture for an average of ten full semesters, or four years. They are not accepted by an Acupuncture college unless they have completed at least two full years in an accredited academic setting, preferably with emphasis of study in the health fields. After completion of academic and clinical courses and completing a national exam, they are eligible for licensing in the state in which they choose to practice.

In some states, a license is issued if a student has completed only 200 hours of study and holds another medical degree, such as Doctor of Chiropractic or Medical Doctor. These practitioners do not read pulses, but simply insert needles into points to relieve pain. In China, they were once called Barefoot Doctors, and often practiced their trade in areas where thoroughly trained Acupuncturists were not available. Treatment by these practitioners may be fine for symptom relief, but it will not balance the system or guarantee cure of the cause of the symptoms.

If this method of acupuncture sounds much like Western drug treatment, it is because it is somewhat similar. A well-trained Barefoot Doctor will do no harm, and your headache will probably be relieved. But if the cause is deep-seated, further treatment may be indicated. And much like Western drug treatment, after the same points are needled many times, treatment may cease to be effective.

When you choose an acupuncturist, ask if they have completed the requirements for practicing at the master level, or if they simply insert needles for relief of pain or discomfort. You must decide whether you wish long-time balance, or quick relief. A master Acupuncturist is able to relieve pain also, but will probably suggest that you continue treatment until the cause of the pain is discovered and cure is achieved.

How many treatments will I need? Usually, acupuncturists require that your first visit include a complete intake to establish a full assessment of your health. They may then suggest that you begin with six or more weekly treatments, followed by re-assessment. Following your initial sessions, you may need to continue treatment weekly or twice monthly, then monthly, and finally, four or five times yearly for health maintenance.

Acupuncture is not like Western treatment, and each patient is unique. Therefore, the number of required treatments is determined by your rate of healing. Your Acupuncturist will keep you informed of your progress on a consistent basis, and you will plan for treatment together.

How much will acupuncture cost? The cost of acupuncture is comparable to that of counseling or other alternative therapies. Insurance often covers some of the cost of Acupuncture. Since many Acupuncturists practice in holistic health organizations or in Chiropractic offices, and utilize their billing systems, long-term payment plans may be arranged.

HERBAL MEDICINE

Oriental herbal medicine is the latest tool to be added to my bag. At this time, I have been taking herbs for inner balance on a regular basis for just over nine months. My introduction to this method of healing came from my daughter, who is a master acupuncturist and herbalist in the Boston area. She suggested that since I am over sixty and edging toward being elderly, I might take herbal medicine to increase my energy and possibly fend off the ravages of age for a few more years. She was not able to help me, since an herbalist needs to evaluate her patient, then recommend treatment. She informed me that a patient may need to have the medicine adjusted many times before obtaining permanent results. Since we are 2000 miles apart, I was not a candidate for her services.

I located a practitioner of acupuncture and herbal medicine, was evaluated, and began to take a prescribed dried herbal mixture daily. I noticed a difference in energy within a month. I felt less tired, and somewhat more comfortable within myself. I began to sleep more soundly and my digestive and elimination systems seemed to work a bit more smoothly. Since I was at a rather advanced age when I began herbal therapy, and have a long history of immune system weakness and dysfunction, I will probably take herbal medicine in some form for the rest of my life. Herbs will not cause negative side effects, but will continue to support my aging organic systems, and to keep me functioning more optimally.

What is Herbal medicine? Herbs are naturally growing plants and other living organisms which contain medicinal, or healing properties. These healing properties may be contained in the leaves, stems or roots of the plant. Chinese herbal medicine may also include parts of sea and land animals. Every country in the world has healing plants growing in its fields and woods and beside its streams and rivers. Herbalists have gathered plants and extracted medicines from them since man began to forage for food. If you have read any of the novels by Jean Auel (Clan of the Cave Bear, etc.) you will have been exposed to stories referring to those peoples who founded herbal medicine. Because every country has its indigenous herbs, every country also has those dedicated herbalists who have learned to extract medicines from plants and use them for healing.

When you are evaluated by a Doctor of Oriental Medicine, he will ask you many questions regarding your health, then take your pulses (see Acupuncture), assess the sound of your voice, evaluate your color and read your tongue. Oriental physicians rely on information they obtain from these procedures to give them a complete picture of the system's inner and outer health.

Practitioners of Western herbal medicine I have consulted have also asked me questions regarding my health, evaluated my color and recommended herbs according to symptoms discovered.

Because herbs are food, and because they do little harm in most cases, many western herbs are dispensed freely at health food stores and markets. But, because they are also medicine, there has been much talk about regulating them, which would most likely make herbs much more difficult to purchase. I do not believe in regulation, since herbal use is very effective in most cases, and it is a cost-effective method for treating many symptoms with very little negative side effect. I do, however, recommend responsible use of herbs, since they are medicine. There are many references on herbal medicines and their safe use, and many proprietors of health food stores are able to recommend research on herbal use.

How do I find the best herbs for me? Unfortunately, only a few countries still have organized systems for prescribing and dispensing herbal medicine. In the west years ago, herbal medicine held a highly respected place in the healing community. But as use of the Western allopathic system of healing increased, herbal medicine began to take a back seat to more aggressive Western medications. There are still many people who grow and utilize western herbs, but aside from courses given in those few colleges which train Naturopathic Physicians or Five-Element Acupuncturists, there is no nationally approved or licensed program to assure those who are seeking treatment for the first time that they are working with a trained, trustworthy practitioner.

Often, the herbal medicine practitioners in this country have been trained by herbalists who teach information which has been passed on to them for many generations. These healers have a reputation which has been confirmed by patients who are satisfied with treatment. When seeking healing treatment using Western herbs, I recommend seeking an herbalist who has an established reputation for herbal dispensation and healing.

Many acupuncturists are also licensed Doctors of Oriental Medicine, and as such are thoroughly trained in the use of Chinese herbal medicine. Herbalists trained in the traditional Chinese manner base their diagnosis on individual patterns and unique disease symptomatology. They realize that diagnosis must be made according to each individual's signs, symptoms and constitution. Information gained through reading the tongue and taking the pulses provides the Chinese herbalist with excellent clues regarding the nature of his patient's overall condition. Herbs obtained from China are strictly regulated and dispensed, so usually prove very reliable. An herbal prescription is formulated for each patient, often consisting of over 20 herbs, mixed to balance the patient's particular makeup. As the patient becomes more balanced, the herbal mixture may be adjusted accordingly.

HOMEOPATHY

The use of homeopathic medicine is not currently popular in this country, mainly due to our scientific method of thought. Scientists can find no reason why homeopathy works. Since they cannot solve this problem, they have largely chosen to ignore it. Other countries including France, Great Britain, Germany and India utilize it everywhere; you can walk into almost any French "Pharmacia" and find a person who has been trained in homeopathic healing to recommend remedies for whatever ails you.

While my husband and I were traveling in France and Germany years ago, he contracted a serious cold. We consulted a homeopathic healer at a local Pharmacia and came away with three remedies which were formulated for his exact symptoms. After taking them according to her specific directions for two days, he was feeling fit and ready to continue traveling. That experience convinced me that it does work when used correctly, so I have chosen to include it in this primer.

What is homeopathy? "Homios" in Greek means similar, and "pathos" means suffering. The idea behind homeopathy is to find an herbal or other "remedy" which acts in a *similar* way to the symptom the patient is experiencing, or *suffering*. When miniscule amounts of this substance are ingested, the body utilizes this miniscule, basically negative invasion to begin a healing process, essentially battling like with like. It is almost the same principle used behind injection with a serum to ward off illness, such as smallpox. A tiny dose of smallpox vaccine is injected under the skin and the body develops antibodies against it, which are then employed to fight the full-fledged disease when the person is exposed to it.

The problem with understanding homeopathy is that the dosages of the herbs and other substances used by homeopathic practitioners are so tiny that even the most powerful scientific microscopes and blood tests cannot detect them in the body. What is even more difficult to understand is that the smaller the dose, the more effective the remedy seems to be. Therefore, according to Western scientists, since these doses are undetectable, they must not exist.

The principle of homeopathy is called the "Law of Similars". This principle has been described by Hippocrates, and was used by the Mayans, the Chinese and Native American cultures. It was Samuel Hahnemann, however, who finally established this Law of Similars as a systematic medical science in the late eighteenth century. Hahnemann found an article written about the treatment of malaria. By using the herbs mentioned in the article, he discovered that when he administered very small doses of these herbs to himself, they caused minor symptoms of malaria. His conclusion was that these tiny doses of herbs must cure malaria as a vaccine does, by producing symptoms which are then fought off by reactions of the body's immune system. Hahnemann continued to use himself as a guinea pig, ingesting substances which caused symptoms of other diseases, and noted that the smaller the doses, the more quickly he became symptom-free. He then began to treat patients using this method, and discovered that they did well.

Why don't we use homeopathy more in this country? Aside from the fact that scientists are not able to detect substances in the remedies, they also do not accept the philosophy of most Homeopathic practitioners, since classically oriented practitioners firmly oppose the use of conventional drugs, stating that they suppress symptoms of disease and the immune system for the most part.

It is the philosophy of the homeopathic doctor that when disease is contracted and a Western medicine is ingested, often the symptoms of the disease seem to disappear. However, once the medication is discontinued, symptoms may return in a more severe form, indicating that the cause of the disease is still present. homeopathic practitioners believe that with ingestion of the correct remedies, the causes of disease are eliminated, resulting in greatly improved inner health and balance.

Orthodox physicians in this country do not accept the suppression theory, and for the most part refuse to acknowledge that miniscule undetectable doses of herbs and other substances are able to eliminate disease. Scientists in Europe, however, decided to integrate homeopathic care centuries ago, and to incorporate the classic homeopathic philosophy along with treatment with Western medicine. There, it is thought that the two types of medicine work well together. Europeans tend to take Homeopathic remedies first, and if they are not effective enough, will supplement them with Western care.

In the early 1900s homeopathy was well respected in America. There were many homeopathic colleges and hospitals. Shortly after the turn of the century, the American Medical Association became increasingly effective in banning it. Because good homeopathic care demands a longer period of one on one with each patient, it was deemed non-cost-effective. Homeopathic practitioners who were also Western physicians could join the newly formed American Medical Association (AMA) only if they agreed to stop their practice of homeopathy. Homeopathic colleges were given poor reports, and as a result they lost students. Within a few decades homeopathy became a lost practice in this country.

How do I locate a Homeopathic practitioner? This is not always an easy task. Homeopathy is a gentle form of treatment for disease, since there is very little danger of side effects from the ingestion of weak doses of a Homeopathic remedy. If it works, it works; if it is not the correct remedy, it does not interact with your system. Note, however, that the more potent dosages of remedies may cause serious side effects if not prescribed properly. Health food stores do not usually supply remedies with more than 12x strength, for this reason. Remedies with stronger effect must be prescribed by a trained Homeopathist.

Because of the ease of obtaining and using lower dose remedies, however, anyone who has the money to buy a Materia Medica, the large book explaining which doses to take for each symptom, and a few bottles of basic remedies can "prescribe" Homeopathic medicine. Training in and licensing for Homeopathic practitioners is fairly loose in most states, since it is not at present a nationally recognized treatment modality. There are, however, many Naturopathic physicians, Chiropractors, Nutritionists and other fully qualified practitioners who have been trained in the administration of Homeopathic remedies.

I suggest you check carefully with any practitioner to assure yourself that they have been fully trained in the dispensing of remedies. The most qualified practitioner is a Homeopathic Physician. Physicians may have been trained in India or Great Britain, since Homeopathy thrives in each of those areas, and there are many accredited colleges. According to my research, there are about 1000 licensed Homeopathic physicians in this country, as well as just over a thousand health care workers who have been fully trained as Homeopathic practitioners.

Can I use the remedies I find in health food stores? I heartily recommend these remedies to give you an idea how Homeopathic medicine reacts in your system. Read the labels carefully, and choose those remedies which most closely match your symptoms. There are mixtures of remedies sold today, which are labeled "cold", "stress" or "allergy", etc. These contain several remedies mixed to match symptoms experienced by most. Certainly they are not prescribed to fit you exactly, but you will discover that most of them relieve symptoms quickly, so long as you choose those most closely resembling your condition.

Taking the wrong remedy will usually cause no harm. I owned a health food store for a short time, and the parents who treated their children's colds and flu with Homeopathic remedies stated that they were often far more effective and quicker than repeated visits to the pediatrician. The children regained energy quickly and their appetites were better.

If you have a deep-seated chronic condition, you will need to seek out a Homeopathic Physician, who will take an extensive history and prescribe the exact remedy you need for the most effective healing results

What else do I need to know about taking remedies? Many remedies do not work when you ingest them after drinking coffee or taking something containing mint. Practitioners also recommend that you do not touch the remedies, but shake a recommended dosage into the cap of the container and tip them into your mouth. They are then placed sub-lingually (under the tongue) until dissolved.

How much does Homeopathic care cost? Remedies are very inexpensive. They come in tubes or small bottles, and are encased in a sugar base. You take the dosage prescribed on the container. If you do not have results after five or six doses, it is probably the wrong remedy. A full Homeopathic evaluation is comparable in cost to that of an acupuncturist or herbist, and usually takes between one and two hours. Some trained Homeopathic providers offer a reduced rate or will present a sliding scale for payment.

CHIROPRACTIC

I bent over to change the sheets on my bed one morning, and could not straighten up. Spasms of pain shot through my lower back and down my right leg. A woman friend who lived with us was seeing a Chiropractic Physician or Chiropractor, for chronic lower back pain. I decided to seek care with this diminutive woman who placed me on large tables which shifted and moved to "adjust" my back. That was my induction into Chiropractic care. I have been treated by a Chiropractor on a fairly regular basis for almost twenty years. I have also experienced treatment for sore shoulders, displaced ribs and stiff neck.

Prior to my experience with this form of care I had visited my primary care physician when my back was "out". He did not believe in Chiropractic, and prescribed strong pain medication and bedrest for ten days. I recovered, but lost valuable work time and felt drugged and incapable of taking care of my children for days after recovery. Following Chiropractic care I did need to take over the counter anti-inflammatory medication and put ice and heat on my back alternately, but I was essentially drug-free and back to work after six treatments.

When I was in high school, I recall my father "sneaking out" to see a Chiropractor following a back injury during a softball game. He had been in bed for days, in pain, and needed to go back to work. He swore my mother and me to secrecy and saw the only Chiropractor he could find, 25 miles away in the next state. He didn't want us to tell because our doctor was a relative and would be appalled that Dad had disobeyed his orders and left his bed to see a quack. Following his second treatment, Dad was feeling fine and returned to work.

What is Chiropractic? Chiropractic is a natural healing system based on the premise that when the nervous system and the spinal column are healthy, the body is much more able to ward off and fight the disease process. The spinal cord has 31 pairs of nerves radiating from the backbone or spinal column. The bones of the spine protect these delicate nerves and provide support for our upright positioning. When these nerves become irritated due to improper positioning of the spinal bones, pain occurs. The Doctor of Chiropractic re-aligns these improper positionings, or treats existing lesions called subluxations to ensure a healthy pain-free spine, and believes that this is the key to an overall healthy system.

Doctors of Chiropractic do not use drugs or surgery. They recommend regular Chiropractic care along with a good supplemented diet. If other treatments are indicated, the Chiropractor will recommend that you consult a medical or other health professional for specific treatment.

Why would I see a Chiropractor? Chiropractic care is sought for many reasons. Usually the first visit occurs because you have been injured, or have strained nerves and muscles in your back and are in pain. You may continue to see a Chiropractor after you are free of pain to maintain health in the spinal and nervous systems. Some Chiropractors have been criticized for recommending regular visits following achievement of freedom from pain. Critics say they "are always going to the Chiropractor, even when they don't need it". Many Chiropractors believe that these visits are necessary for pain prevention and continued spinal maintenance.

What may I expect with my first visit? The Chiropractic physician will usually conduct a thorough examination during your first visit. They will take x-rays of your back and neck, as well as a thorough medical history. They will then test reflexes, take blood pressure, weight and pulse and do a complete structural examination, emphasizing the spine, extremities and musculoskeletal system.

Following this, the Chiropractor will evaluate your condition and probably administer a spinal "adjustment". This involves the use of one or more of a number of methods to begin to bring the condition of your spine back to normal alignment. Following this adjustment, the Chiropractor may recommend massage or ultrasound treatment, which will deepen and speed up the healing process.

What methods may be used for adjustments? The most frequent method employed by Chiropractors is a direct adjustment, which is accomplished by the doctor placing hands on your back or neck or hips and quickly re-positioning the vertebra which is out of place. This is often called "cracking" the back or neck, because of the sound it produces. It is not painful, but the sound may cause discomfort in a patient.

Other methods of adjustment include use of a device which looks somewhat like a staple gun, called an Activator. The Chiropractor places you face-down on a table and determines which vertebrae are out of line with a series of arm and leg movements; they then place the Activator against the effected vertebra and jolt it. This causes no discomfort. A third treatment method is called Counter-strain. The Chiropractor places a fingertip on either side of an effected vertebra and gently presses or manipulates until they feel change in the area. This is the most gentle and comfortable form of Chiropractic I have experienced, but I needed extra treatment to achieve total freedom from pain.

Some Chiropractors achieve direct adjustment by using a table which drops in the middle. They will place you on this table in a position where the affected vertebrae need treatment, then drop the table slightly, jolting the back into place. Other tables move the lower back in a figure eight motion, gently re-aligning discs which have been misplaced.

Which form of treatment would you recommend? I have experienced all of the above forms of Chiropractic, administered by many doctors, and have found them all quite effective. I have also learned that Chiropractors usually employ the type of treatment with which they are most comfortable. It is up to you to choose the method which suits you. Because Chiropractors are human, and therefore behave humanly, they will sometimes work to convince you that their way is best. They believe this, of course, and it is best for them. But you are not your Chiropractor, and you must search until you discover the treatment method which works for you.

I do recommend that you be wary of those treatment plans which involve more sessions than you require for spinal health. Following initial treatment, make sure your Chiropractor and you agree on a number of future visits. You do not need to be coerced into signing a plan which may cost hundreds of dollars per year and keep you coming back for an unnecessary number of visits. If you have insurance, make sure you know how many visits are covered so you don't have to incur unnecessary expense. You know you are maintaining well when your back feels good most of the time, and you don't need to run back for treatment because you are in spasm. Treatment is a personal thing, and each case is different.

How much will Chiropractic care cost? Most insurance plans will cover some Chiropractic care. If yours does not, check with your Chiropractor; they may offer a treatment plan for a reduced fee. If fee for service is a problem for you, you may want to search around, since some Chiropractors may offer lower-priced treatment plans. For example, a Chiropractor who practices from home may offer services for less than one who has a plush office.

Note: Since Chiropractors are invested in the health of their clients' whole systems, they may offer services beyond simply adjusting you. Some are also nutritionists, or offer herbal or Homeopathic medications, or even Acupressure,

Cranio-sacral treatment, Reiki or Acupuncture. Although most of these practitioners are fully trained in a complementary practice, care is needed to make sure you receive proper treatment in all areas. You may need to check to assure yourself that your Chiropractor has received proper training in any alternative practice they offer.

For example, training to become a fully trained Acupuncturist is a very intensive process. But many states will issue a license to a practitioner who has had only 200 hours of training in acupuncture. These practitioners may be able to treat simple physical ailments (in China they call them Barefoot Doctors) such as headache or shoulder pain, but they are not qualified enough in the use of needles to completely balance the physical/mental system.

Ask your Chiropractor about qualifications before you commit to treatment other than Chiropractic adjustments. Arm yourself with knowledge of the hours or years it takes to qualify as a nutritionist, herbalist or acupuncturist. Research in advance allows you to obtain optimal available treatment.

EXERCISE

I have a friend in her mid-seventies who walks, swims and lifts weights daily, and takes yoga and aerobics classes twice weekly. I am not making this up. Just thinking of her schedule exhausts me. I hate to exercise. I know it and everyone who knows me, knows it. Years ago when I studied cultural eating patterns through the ages, I discovered that I was the Cold-climate type. This body type is built solid, close to the ground and chunky, because we need to sit for long periods of time in weather which is too cold for normal life functioning, and we need to be able to store large amounts of fat to protect us from the cold, and to survive when the food supply is lean. We are able to go for long times without eating, and can put away large quantities of food during a meal. Little exercise, two to three large meals daily, slow-moving, with an energy level that is not adapted for running or rushing around constantly, but is enduring. That's me. It's not only me, but it was true for every female member of my family on my father's side. All of the women were large, slow-moving and hated exercise.

My mother's family were the opposite. Long, lean bones, streamlined energetic bodies, the need to eat many small meals daily rather than three larger ones. This body type was adapted for warm dry climates, where little clothing was needed, food was in constant supply, people were always on the move. The meals my mother prepared were sparse, since she preferred to eat often. She would walk miles each day, and eat a handful of nuts or some cheese when she came home. My father and I were always hungry after meals, so we would forage for sweets late at night. We were both considerably overweight.

My body is not the one preferred by today's society. Current media has informed us that our bodies need to be long, lean and toned. Those of us who have bought this media message spend our spare time consumed with eating little and exercising lots, striving to achieve correct Body Mass Index, consuming low-carbohydrate diets, meals with more protein and less harmful fats. We join gyms in huge numbers, jog, swim and lift our way to perfect abs and pecs and quads. Most of us do not consider whether we are enjoying ourselves while we whittle our bodies like chunks of wood to the shapes they are supposed to be; we do it because we have been led to think that it must be right, since it is the accepted thing.

Then, there are those who have decided you cannot afford these programs, or do not enjoy spending hours each week assuring yourself that you meet a standard set by a group of people you will never encounter. You choose instead to sit around, eat whatever beckons to you and continue to grow fat, often to the point where you lose your health.

I was the latter for much of my adult life. I would half-heartedly exercise for a week or two; I bought 5 or 6 of those machines which were guaranteed to give me a lovely shape within weeks and used each of them for a week; I joined each new exercise class which was offered, and attended them for an average of three visits. I finally gave up, deciding that exercise was not for me and never would be. I sold my machines, cancelled memberships in classes and gyms and spent my spare time reading, watching tv and snacking, poking fun at infomercials advertising the latest new exercise fad, and spreading out like Jabba the Hut.

By the time I was in my late fifties, I was flabby, often out of breath and almost fifty pounds overweight. I had a knee replaced five years earlier and was becoming worried that it would not support my weight. My diet was not extremely unbalanced due to the work I had accomplished to date, but it contained far too many calories for my size and lack of activity.

I began to research types of exercise, and finally formulated a program of exercise I could work with. I feel it is important that you do what you want to do, because the will does not take kindly to being pushed into movement which it does not enjoy.

What is exercise? Exercise is any activity which requires physical or mental exertion, especially when it involves the idea of keeping the system fit. When your body is physically fit, it is responsive, feels light, moves easily and feels healthy. If you want to know how total fitness looks, watch a child of four or five. She will run, climb, twist, bend and move with complete ease, so long as she is of normal size and weight for her age.

So what happens to the child who compromises her fitness? She learns to ride instead of walk, eats too much, plays too little, restricts her movements too much, sits too long. By the time she is a young adult, she may be overweight, sluggish, feel tired much of the time, develop joint or digestive problems or have a feeling of general malaise. Fitness improves when she remembers to exercise as she did when she was young. If you begin a program to regain or maintain fitness while you are younger, most of the movement you have lost can be regained. The longer you wait, the more difficult it is to regain or maintain a fit body. But do not let that stop you, since every step you take toward total fitness brings you one step further from your couch potato days.

What are the various types of exercise? There are certainly many exercise methods which help you increase strength, improve circulation and burn fat or convert it to muscle. A few are listed below, and information to research them can be found in the Resources section of this book.

Aerobic exercises are those which increase heart action and circulation, and are great for cardio-vascular strength. Care needs to be used when doing aerobic exercise, since there may be too much stress on ankle, knee and hip joints when they are overused, and problems when you are older may result. Less stressful exercises of this type include water aerobics and use of mini-trampolines.

Resistance exercise builds muscle strength and size, and burns fat. Weight lifting, isometrics, use of resistance weights in a pool are all helpful. Resistance exercise using weights needs planning, since different groups of muscles need to be targeted, and it is not good to strain the muscles on a daily basis. Resistance exercise utilizing breathwork and isometric movements may be done whenever you have a few moments, and are very successful when repeated over the course of a few months.

Stretching is just what it states, a series of planned movements to stretch the muscles and increase range of motion and circulation. Yoga for exercise, Tai chi and Pilates are all excellent stretching modalities.

Walking remains the cheapest, best all-round exercise you can do. Whether done briskly when it is aerobic, or in a meandering way, which moves lymph and increases circulation, it is always better to walk than to sit. I become easily bored with a regular walking regimen, although I meander regularly through malls or down city streets, and I thoroughly enjoy a long hike with my dog once or twice a month.

Breathing. There is also another type of exercise which involves inner body rather than outer body movement. This exercise works with the breath. When you breathe in deeply, slowly let the breath out, then hold the stomach in for 10 seconds you will burn calories, increase your lung capacity and in time strengthen your abdominal muscles.

How much exercise is enough? One of the "rules for exercise" which puts me off is the statement that we need at least an hour of vigorous movement three times a week to make a difference in our health. I do not believe this for one minute. If you have not been exercising at all, and you decide you are willing to move five minutes a day, two days a week, it is far better to move for ten minutes a week than to continue to watch tv and eat because you are not willing to move for three hours weekly. If you push yourself to exercise according to another's rules, you may soon find yourself back on the couch. Contract a small change for yourself, then carry it through. No matter how small the change is, it will be for the better, since you will take a small step toward deeper balance and more robust health.

I strongly recommend you experiment with those exercise regimens which are best for your personal health, and most enjoyed by your body/mind. Gyms often offer one or two free visits; take advantage of them, and if you are not comfortable after a few visits, move on to something else. Send away for video programs which offer a 30 day free trial; I don't feel the least uncomfortable sending them back if I don't like them. Pieces of machinery often are sold with the same 30-day guarantee; try them, you may like one. It is important that we move, but it is more important that we enjoy the movement. This is the only thing which will allow exercise to work for us.

Which exercises do you like? Convinced that movement was necessary for me, and knowing that change is as difficult for me as it is for everyone, I was afraid I could never stay with a program of exercise long enough to do myself any good. I finally decided to follow the advice I often gave my clients. I would stop worrying about what I weighed; instead, I would concentrate on becoming as healthy and physically strong as I could be. I decided there must be a program out there for one who hates exercise, a regimen I could enjoy enough to stick with for more than a few weeks.

I must confess it took me years of experimentation and failure to discover the right combination of movement modalities for myself. I also confess that what I do now may not last forever, but today, I enjoy the things I do to get myself moving. Swimming is my favorite exercise. I love the water, but regular swimming taxes my shoulders and lower back, so I could not stay in the pool long enough to reap full benefit from my swim. When I discovered an exercise belt I could use in the pool I was ecstatic. I found mine in a catalogue, but pool supply shops carry a number of styles. Belted safely in, I developed a half-hour routine which supplies enough movement to burn off fat.

Therapeutic yoga was the second exercise tool I discovered. Yoga teachers have developed programs to help you stretch no matter how disabled you may be. You work at your own speed, and within your unique circumstances. Practice three times weekly for a half hour, and you soon discover your range of movement increasing, and your balance becoming more solid. Yoga has gained greatly in popularity in the past few years, and classes are available in almost every community.

Breathwork for toning is the third tool in my exercise bag. There are now many programs which will train you to breathe deeply while you do simple resistance exercises. This is my substitute for weight training, which I respect but abhor. Fifteen minutes twice a week has toned my abdomen and decreased my expanse by a couple of inches.

The fourth tool I use is a video tape for modified Pilates. This is a series of 10-15 simple exercises done on the floor or on a Massage table which target increase in strength of the abdominal muscles. I found the video I use on the internet, but there are many programs available now, since it is also a popular exercise regimen.

Would you recommend exercise for weight loss? Definitely; and it is even more important for maintaining weight loss. As I have stated, I abhorred exercise, so I decided at first to approach weight loss with reduction of caloric intake. I eliminated 400 calories a day from my diet, and ate less oil and fat, and more protein. I lost 10 pounds in a fairly short time, then stopped short. No matter how little I ate, how careful I was, the pounds would not come off. I feared the worst; I would need to resort to EXERCISE.

Those of you who have followed strict diet regimens for years are all too aware that they work very well for a while. You are able to lose up to 50 pounds or more in a year, depending on the amount you need to lose, if you follow these programs strictly, every day. But many of you realize that when you become bored with the strict diet, and decide to return to your original way of eating, the pounds begin to pile on at an alarming rate, due to the fact that your body's metabolism, the mechanism for burning calories, has been severely compromised by the consistent reduction in caloric intake, especially if daily exercise has not been included in your program.

Permanent weight loss is an elusive concept. Only 3-5% of those who diet are able to achieve it. I need to share with you that there is only one way to get there. You need to permanently reduce your caloric intake, and plan to exercise moderately each day of your life. When you truly know that this is a lifetime commitment, and not a quick diet to get you to your 20th reunion without that extra 15 pounds, or to fit into that bikini next summer, you will succeed.

Having said this, I stick by what I said earlier regarding the amount of exercise you need. Knowing that you need to exercise so much to lose weight may send you back to the couch. But, if you increase your exercise a bit each week or month you will begin to feel better and look better, and what is more important, you will begin to discover your authentic self. The authentic self is never sick. She may not be thin, or physically beautiful according to society's standards, but she is healthy and real, and this makes her beautiful to herself, and to others. Your compromised self may desire thinness because it helps you to be more accepted; your authentic self wants health because she needs to accept herself fully. She is not invested in achieving physical perfection to gain the acceptance of others.

If your health is being compromised by severe overweight, and you need to remove pounds to improve this condition, by all means find a program which will help you. But while you are following this program, I recommend that you seek the tools you need to keep you on your path to wellness. When you receive counseling and possibly Acupuncture, Herbal medicine or Homeopathy along with your strict weight loss regimen, you gain access to your authentic self much more quickly, and gain the emotional strength to maintain your health once the weight is off.

Did you lose weight with your exercise program? Yes, I have lost some. I have not yet reached the weight which the calculated Body Mass Index (BMI) states is best for me, but I have reached more peace with myself, a greater degree of health and balance and a definite weight loss, which I am able to maintain. I also continually work to re-think my original expectations, and to become a better friend to my body, my self. Pushing weight around with constant ups and downs is not a good way to treat the body. Thinking health instead of thinness and working steadily toward this is a much more caring way to treat the home you live in.

BODYWORK

Counseling, nutrition, acupuncture and Chiropractic care were the four tools in my bag for many years. I assumed that if I ate a fairly healthy diet, saw a therapist when I felt it necessary, attended to my sore back when it barked at me and scheduled regular Acupuncture treatments to keep my energy balanced I was surely taking care of all of my health needs. Ten years ago I met a massage therapist who convinced me otherwise. I had experienced massage for relaxation periodically, and considered the process a treat with which to pamper myself when I needed it.

With this new massage therapist, I felt very different. Following our session, I was very emotional, and felt as if I had rid myself of a burden. He had worked with massage, Acupressure and Foot Reflexology to "unknot" my muscles, and release energy trapped within them. He told me that although it is fine to release negative emotion and change patterns which do not work for us in counseling, it is also important to attend to the energy trapped in the physical body. This energy is often held very tightly in the lymph system, muscles and nerves, and nothing will release it short of direct manipulation of the muscle groups.

I soon adopted bodywork as another tool which would help peel off more layers into my authentic self. I realized as I experienced work on my body that there is much memory held on a cellular level. The mind is fine for helping to work out those psychological "knots" which are contained in our consciousness. However, there is a mountain of information contained in those parts of us which remain unconscious. Each of our cells contains a minuscule file of memories. These are stored in the form of energy. When the body is stimulated on a cellular level, cells are able to release these memories, which frees the energy to be used in more productive ways.

For example, if you feel a need to weep during a massage session, and allow yourself to cry, grief is released into your consciousness. You may suddenly remember a sad time, and are able to release this memory from those cells which have held it. The energy you release then goes to other cells which are responsible for the body's greater health. These "health" cells may be depleted, due to lack of energy. When the body moves energy from negative holdings to depleted areas, depletion dissipates, and you feel lighter, more energized.

I researched different forms of bodywork and decided to experiment with the ones included below. I have experienced many forms of massage, Acupressure, Reflexology, Craniosacral Therapy, Reiki, Therapeutic Touch and Externally Transmitted Qigong. All have helped me to relax, release inner stress, alleviate chronic pain and feel clearer and more energetic. I later became a Reiki master/ teacher and learned Qigong breathwork in order to help my counseling clients to feel deeper balance.

I realize that this is a very foreign concept for many of you. If you need an exercise to demonstrate the movement of energy, try this: next time you have a frontal headache, sit in a comfortable chair and place your feet flat on the floor. Place the first two fingers of your right hand just between your eyebrows. Place your left hand on your lower abdomen, just below your navel. Take ten deep breaths, and ask the energy from your headache to go to your lower abdomen. (This is the center of the body's energy, and can always use an extra dose of energy). This is also good for feelings of frustration. Your headache will usually dissipate in a very short time, leaving you more calm and centered.

What is bodywork? Bodywork can be a form of exercise, since most bodywork increases circulation, stretches muscles and involves deep breathing. But bodywork as a whole is a more passive way of working with the physical system. I like to think of exercise as movement I initiate, and bodywork as movement initiated by another with my full consent. During a Bodywork session, a practitioner works with you to improve and heal your body/mind. The worker's task is to stir up and stimulate your inner healing energy through direct or indirect contact or touch; yours is to allow yourself to receive and relax, allowing change to occur. When you allow another's energy to work with yours, change often occurs quickly and on a deep level. Allowing caring touch during massage often produces a relaxation response which is impossible when you work alone to effect physical change.

Bodywork is often called energy work. The term "energy" may be difficult for some to understand. The word energy is often misinterpreted when applied to work with the body. Some consider energy that which they feel when they are able to accomplish a lot, to keep moving. That is one way to interpret energy, but since it is everywhere, it can be understood differently in each situation. Energy is basically *life force*, and is contained in all living things.

Each person has his own unique energy system. Some are very fast movers, others are slower but have much endurance. Both are fine, and both have the potential to be optimally healthy. When you try to change your basic energy system, disease often occurs. Those who are meant to move more slowly may think it best if they push themselves. Their endurance suffers from this, and they become overly fatigued. Those who are able to move constantly are fatigued when they ask their systems to slow down. It takes more energy for them to live slowly, since it is not a natural thing.

It is the philosophy of those who work with the body that each person's unique energy is able to be moved, manipulated and finally changed when pockets of it become dammed up, or when it becomes depleted in certain areas. When inner energy is flowing smoothly, balance is easier to achieve.

Because the purpose of bodywork is to effect change, and because change is difficult and we are choosing to change with help from outside, a deep trust needs to exist between you and your Bodyworker. Those who are uncomfortable with direct touch often avoid this type of healing work, fearing that a practitioner may cause physical harm, or an emotional or sexual reaction, or that she may judge or criticize the body. If you have issues with touch, you may choose to begin bodywork with a non-invasive relaxation and healing technique, such as Reiki.

A well-trained, experienced Bodyworker will explain technique before you receive a session. They will allow you to question them, and will work with you to alleviate fears. They will not force a procedure on you without first explaining it fully and receiving your consent. As in counseling, you often are able to interview the Bodyworker before commitment to a session. You need to feel comfortable about the technique and the provider before receiving the work. If you are not, if you feel pushed or rushed into the work, feel free to leave.

Bodywork is becoming more popular in the past few years, since it is non-verbal, relaxing and beneficial in a relatively short period of time. It is a great relief from the rush of today's business world to come to a quiet, serene space where candles are burning, soft music is playing, the scent of aromatic incense hovers in the air and lavender-scented oils are gently rubbed on your back. All of this, and you need only receive it without conversation. More and more, businesses are providing a space for Bodyworkers in their facilities, to aid in relief of mental and physical stress for this heavily burdened society.

Often, clients receive bodywork in conjunction with other forms of healing work such as counseling, acupuncture or Chiropractic. As deep emotion is released, and as mental patterns change, the body often holds on to negative patterns with a deeper resistance. Body work in conjunction with counseling often speeds the process of healing, allowing the body to release and relax.

What are some of the types of bodywork? I like to place bodywork into two categories: contact-related and non-invasive. Contact-related bodywork involves direct touch in the form of rubbing, poking, holding etc. between the practitioner and the client. Non-invasive work involves the client sitting or lying fully clothed on a table, while the practitioner works either lightly touching the body or head, or often some inches above the body. Included here are short descriptions of methods of work in each category. I have chosen to include only those types of body work which I have experienced personally. As I have stated before, this is my path; you may choose to travel a totally separate road to healing.

I have listed other forms of bodywork in the Resources section of this book. Please feel free to explore. It often takes many trials to find just the right combination of work for your unique body.

Contact-related bodywork.

Therapeutic Massage, in which the muscles are stretched in various ways to release toxins trapped within, allow lymphatic fluids to move more easily, relax chronically tight areas and alleviate pain, is a very common form of direct contact bodywork. There are many types of massage which range from deep or therapeutic manipulation to gentle relaxation and stretching of the muscle systems. Massage therapists may utilize hot packs, vibrators, hot rocks or other devices to release and relax the body. Massage usually takes place on a table, where you lie nude or partially clothed, draped with a sheet covering all of the body except the part being worked on. Most states require licensing for massage; if a practitioner does not openly display their license, you may ask them for a state number or the school in which they were trained. Therapists who are not licensed may not be fully trained, or may offer non-professional services such as sexual massage.

Unplanned sexual response during a session is often a fear which keeps a client from receiving massage. Licensed Therapeutic Massage practitioners are fully trained to deal with a client's sexual response during massage. They will not act on it, and will assure that the client does not feel uncomfortable. The frontal torso is almost never massaged, except with full permission of the client, and only in situations where necessity calls for it. The therapist will massage the limbs, the back, the shoulders and neck, and in some cases, the face and head. Full body massage usually takes one hour, and half hour massages may be offered for localized problems such as lower back or tight neck and shoulders.

The massage practitioner may offer to come to your home, or to your office with a table. They may provide fully clothed back massage using a special chair for that purpose. Be prepared to spend more for your session when your practitioner comes to you. Back massages may be offered in public places such as malls for as little as a dollar per minute. This is a wonderful introduction to direct touch, and allows you to meet the therapist before committing yourself to full body massage.

Acupressure is another common form of contact related bodywork. The practitioner is trained to press or rub places on the body called "points". These points ore often tender or sore, since they indicate dammed-up energy which has gathered in pathways in the body called "meridians". To receive acupressure you often lie on a table, or the practitioner may treat you in a seated or standing position. You may be asked to disrobe and don a loose gown, or you may be treated fully clothed. Acupressure practitioners may also stimulate points with a device which emits a slight electronic current which enters the skin and breaks up blockages. A session with an acupressure practitioner takes about an hour, and the cost is similar to a massage session.

Reflexology of the hands and feet is often used in conjunction with therapeutic Massage and acupressure. The Reflexologist stimulates inner energy by deeply massaging areas of the whole foot or hand. The philosophy behind this practice is that there are certain areas of the hands and feet that correspond to organs and sections of the body. When these areas are deeply massaged, healing occurs within the body.

Cranio/Sacral Therapy is a fairly new system which stems from research done at the turn of the century concerning the movement of the bones of and fluid surrounding the skull and spine, and the relationship of this movement to the movement patterns in the rest of the body. The CST practitioner uses a very light touch to test for restrictions in the cranio/sacral system, monitoring the rhythm of the cerebrospinal fluid as it flows through the system. With light touch, they then assist the hydraulic forces in the cranio/sacral system to flow more freely, thus improving the body's internal environment. When malfunctions are detected and changed the body's natural ability to self-heal is strengthened.

Other forms of direct touch which balance the physical body include Rolfing, the Alexander Technique, Shiatsu, Zero Balancing and the Feldenkrais Method. All are well-documented forms of systemic balance, and all have been used successfully by many. I have not directly experienced these, but I offer references to some in the Resource section of this book.

Non-invasive bodywork.

Reiki has become a popular form of non-invasive bodywork. During a Reiki session, the client is usually lying prone and fully clothed on a table, although there are situations which call for treatment in a seated or standing position. The Reiki practitioner stands to the side and places the hands lightly on or above the head and body, holding them there until they feel that change in energy has occurred. They are aware of change because the area feels warmer, cooler or sometimes "tingles". Reiki healing is based on moving inner energy through a series of whirling centers which travel through the torso, called Chakras. Chakra energy was discovered in India thousands of years ago. The belief is that there are between six and nine major Chakras, and several minor Chakras in other parts of the body including the hands and feet. Reiki practice originated with a Japanese healer named Usui, who had visions of an ancient Tibetan healing system that had remained dormant for centuries. Thus the Japanese name Reiki, meaning loosely "energy entering".

The Reiki practitioner receives training through certified Reiki Master/Teachers, who supply them with the sacred symbols needed to attune them to energy which travels from outside the system through their hearts, heads and hands. Reiki reached America through Hawaii, and Reiki teachers often are able to trace their healing lineage directly back to Usui. There are three degrees of Reiki healing attunement, called Reiki I, Reiki II and Master Level. The transmitted energy becomes more potent with each degree. Ask your practitioner to tell you which degree they use to heal. Often, Reiki I practitioners opt not to work for monetary exchange, since the level of their energy transmission is lower, and trainees do not receive healing symbols to assist and deepen the transmission of energy. Those who opt to receive only the first level of attunement often wish to use it to heal themselves or their families.

Reiki is always a relaxing treatment, but it often requires consecutive treatments to achieve permanent physical or mental change. Treatments given many days in succession often heal very deeply. Reiki may be used in care facilities such as nursing homes and hospitals, since it is non-invasive and very relaxing. I am a Reiki Master/Teacher, and utilize treatments in conjunction with counseling to achieve deeper and quicker results. Before I began to use Reiki as a relaxing tool following therapy a client might leave a session feeling very emotional. With a short Reiki treatment before leaving, the client feels much more relaxed and prepared to leave.

Reiki practitioners often offer free clinics. Here, two or three practitioners may work on one person. This is a wonderful way to experience bodywork for the first time, since it causes no harm, is very relaxing and is totally non-invasive.

Therapeutic Touch is another form of non-invasive bodywork which also frees blocked energy allowing it to move to the places in the system where it is depleted. The participant may sit in a chair, stand or lie down to receive TT. The practitioner places hands slightly above the head and moves them down the body; they repeat this motion until the energy is evenly distributed. TT practitioners are often invited to nursing homes, hospitals and hospice homes to relieve the anxiety of patients. Many nurses are trained in TT, since they work around those who may benefit from touch, but may not be comfortable with it. Many TT practitioners also certify in Reiki, since they feel that the ability to heal is deepened with this added modality.

Externally Transmitted Qigong. is a third form of non-invasive work. ETQ is often done by practitioners who are trained in Qigong. Qigong, or Chi Kung, is loosely translated as "work with the breath". There are thousands of forms of Qigong, including martial arts such as Karate or Tai Quo Do, gentle movement exercises such as Tai Chi, passive breathwork to heal internally, and externally transmitted forms to heal outside of the self. The practitioner of ETQ may stand next to or quite far from the patient, feeling their energy. They then transmit energy through the hands with a series of meaningful gestures. Practitioners train for many years to direct the energy to the places where it is needed.

There are many other forms of indirect and distance healing available to those who seek deeper inner balance. Some are included in the Resources section. My advice is to read about those which interest you, call a practitioner in your area to obtain further information and experience a session to determine whether this work is right for you. If it helps, go for it If not, feel free to continue your search.

How do I find a bodyworker? There is a national network of licensed therapeutic bodyworkers which is accessible on the internet. You may wish to consult these sites to locate practitioners in your area. Other ways to locate a qualified practitioner include your local Chiropractor, holistic health services, Naturopathic physicians, or word of mouth. Often a health food store will have a bulletin board listing bodywork services provided in your area. Many areas offer an alternative newsletter which contains information regarding local services.

As with any service in which trust is required, be sure that you feel comfortable with a provider before committing to their services. Check their qualifications, visit their places of business, talk with them about treatments and what they will entail. Be sure you are heard if you voice concerns about entering a new type of treatment. It is important that you feel free to refuse treatment if it does not seem right for you.

How often will I need bodywork? As with most alternative therapies, you will probably need a series of treatments in the beginning, to accustom your body to the new method of releasing toxic material. Many practitioners recommend four or five weekly sessions, followed by one session monthly for maintenance. Massage, for example, frees stagnant or stuck lymph fluid in the body, and many practitioners feel that if you wait too long between sessions, this fluid begins to "dam up" again, causing muscle and nerve discomfort. I find that 8-10 sessions yearly keeps me fairly limber. A series of Reiki sessions is often able to measurably strengthen the immune system. Other forms of bodywork may offer the same results. You and your Bodyworker need to decide together the number of treatments which are most beneficial and comfortable for you.

How much will bodywork cost? A qualified Bodyworker may charge as much as other qualified complementary health providers such as Chiropractors or counselors. Providers may offer sliding scale fees for service or other payment plans, such as use of a credit card. Think of the analogy I presented earlier; the fees you pay a good provider will ensure you improved health and a further glimpse into your authentic self, and will likely pay large dividends for years to come.

BREATHWORK (Passive Qigong)

During a workshop toward the end of my training in Psychosynthesis Counseling, I was asked to visualize the ways in which I would utilize my training. Our group was led through a complex visual meditation in which we saw ourselves in the future, and a message was supposedly given to us directing us toward work we would be asked to do. All went well, and I began to visualize my message. It was BREATHE. That's all. Just one word, repeated over and over. I sat with the group of eighteen while they shared the wonderful visions they had concerning their futures. Finally Tom, the leader, asked me if I had anything to share. I hesitated, thinking it was such a small, ridiculous message. It was so obvious; everyone needed to breathe. "All I got was BREATHE", I offered. Most of the group smiled or chuckled. I would have

"You need to pay close attention to that message", Tom said. "I have a feeling it's very important for you."

Ten years later, while bartering energy work with a Tai Chi teacher in Maine I was exposed to the work of Ken Cohen, a major contributor to the acceptance of the Chinese methods of Qigong in the western world. Qigong, loosely translated, means "work with the breath". Cohen teaches that Qigong has many different forms, some of which were mentioned in the Exercise section. Exercise is the active form of Qigong; breathwork is the passive form. During physical exercise, Qigong dictates that the body moves while the mind remains quiet. Passive Qigong requires the mind to move while the body remains quiet. Breathwork, or Passive Qigong, uses the mind to move the breath, and is just as effective as exercise or active Qigong in the body's healing and balancing process.

I used Cohen's exercises intensively every day, read everything he has written, and five years later, began to teach breathing exercises to retirees in my community.

Why is breathwork so important? Count the times you breathe in one minute. Also, notice where your breath comes into your body. If you breathe any more than 8 times a minute, or your breath travels no lower than your chest, your body is not relaxed, and is suffering inner (often unconscious) stress. When the body is unconsciously stressed, energy is not flowing smoothly, lymph is damming up, lungs are not fully expanded, organs and muscles are tense. It takes more energy to keep your immune system healthy when your body is stressed. When breathing is deepened and slowed, the body naturally relaxes. When breath is directed to affected organs or muscles, they relax, let go of toxins and begin to heal. Ten minutes a day of directed breathwork may change the energy flow in your body within a few months.

Who benefits most from breathwork? Breathwork is wonderful for anyone who wants to heal on a passive level, but it is especially helpful for those who are not able to participate in physical exercise due to chronic illness or limited range of motion caused by arthritis or other physically debilitating conditions. Directed breathing exercises are able to relax the system, relieve physical or mental pain, move energy in the body/mind, improve the immune system and raise endorphins to promote a greater sense of well-being.

Within months of regular breathwork participants have demonstrated deeper and slower normal everyday breathing. Most also experienced a heightened sense of well-being and improved circulation, indicated by clearer eyes, younger-looking skin and shinier hair, relief from chronic digestive and elimination problems, and a general feeling of improved health.

How do I learn breathwork? Work with the breath is the least expensive form of healing. It requires no special clothing, no work on a table, no regular monetary outlay, no uncomfortable physical workout, no change in diet. The best way to learn it is to do it. Ken Cohen has many books and tapes available at large bookstores, and tapes and videos are now available by others such as Dr. Andrew Weil. Cohen presents a simple test at the beginning of his teaching to assess your breathing. It consists of four questions: How do you breathe (is the breath shallow? ragged? fast? rapid?) Where does your breath go in your body? What moves when you breathe? How often do you breathe (how many breaths in a minute)? At the beginning of your practice, write the answers to these questions, then ask yourself the same questions every month or so. You discover after a few months that everything has improved, and that you are much more aware of your breath.

Which breathing exercises might be best for me? We all need relief from stress, so I recommend that you do a relaxation breathing at the beginning of each practice session. After that, since you are unique and each exercise is different, you may want to experiment until you find the series of exercises which are right for you. For example, if you have digestive problems, there are breathing exercises directed at the healing of the stomach, spleen, pancreas, gall bladder and liver, and intestines. Choose a few of these daily, do them for five minutes each, and you will soon discover that the energy in this system improves greatly.

You may lie down as you breathe unless you fall asleep easily, when it is recommended that you sit. The diaphragm is more comfortable in a supine position, so I usually do my breathing exercises lying down. If you are a normally active person, standing may be best for you. There are whole books written on the Standing breathing exercise. You just stand, relaxed, gazing with "soft eyes", hands placed loosely by your sides, feet apart, knees slightly bent, and breathe slowly and deeply into your diaphragm for five or more minutes daily. This is a very powerful healing exercise. It seems simple, but often takes some time to do comfortably.

Can breathwork help me lose weight? For many of us, it's all about weight loss. The need to lose weight often brings us into the alternative field of health and healing, since it is so difficult and the use of western medical science seems to have little effect on long-term weight loss and maintenance. Society continually sends us the double message of eat and be thin. If we peruse any magazine we see ads displaying luscious looking food next to articles about the latest weight-loss craze, or recipes for fat-laden foods next to anorexic models displaying the latest fashion. (Be aware that the input of double messages can make you feel crazy!)

The use of breathwork may not directly ensure that you lose lots of pounds, but yes, it will help. More than directly removing weight, breathwork removes the anxieties of carrying extra weight. With regular breathing exercises, you begin to feel more quiet, more content, more comfortable within your body. These exercises will expand your lungs, soothe your digestive system, regulate your energy. When the energy within begins to flow more smoothly, everything in your life flows more smoothly. When life becomes easier to bear, the need to medicate or cover emtions with food diminishes considerably. Therefore, you release the need to overeat, and choose less food and more comfort.

There are many breathwork experts who have developed programs of regulated breathing combined with simple resistance exercises. They claim that large amounts of weight can be lost when their regimens are followed religiously. Tapes and videos are available to teach these programs. As with any other program, persistence and commitment are necessary for positive results. The programs I have used require 15 minutes a day, or 15 minutes every other day for best results.

I used one program three days a week for 6 weeks. My lungs felt larger and my breathing improved, my energy level seemed better, and I felt firmer and more fit. Did I lose weight? No, but I did not gain any. For me at that time, that was a good thing. I stopped the program after the six week period. I surmise that if I had stayed with it, and had been even the least committed to lowering my caloric intake, I might have lost a few pounds. So I do not discount the program as a method to lose weight. I am now thoroughly convinced that once you are committed to weight loss and weight loss maintenance, any program will work for you. And, until that commitment happens for you, no program will work.

MEDITATION

Meditation may be the last tool I am recommending for your bag, but that's only because something needed to be listed last. I consider meditation an extremely valuable tool, and use it daily. This form of relaxing and balancing the body/mind has probably been around since the first human sat entranced before a blossoming flower or a flickering fire, and realized that when he concentrated on this alone for a long period of time, he became calm, balanced, relaxed and focused, and he could transfer these feelings to every area of his life.

There are so many tapes and books on the subject, I hesitate to even add to them. But I will, since this is a primer, and those of you who may have picked it up to peruse it may not be aware of what meditation really is, and how to begin to utilize it.

What is meditation? Meditation sounds like the most simple thing you could think of doing. It merely involves placing yourself in a quiet environment, focusing on one thing or concept and allowing your mind to clear itself of all the flotsam and jetsam which usually float through it. That's it. The idea behind meditation is to relax the body/mind to the point where your brainwaves leave the alpha or wide-awake state and drift to other levels. These levels are beta, delta and gamma. You do not need to worry about which ones are present at what time; you need only to relax, focus and allow your mind to do the rest.

There are those who would make meditation a more complicated process by instruction on how to sit, or what to wear, or what image or word to concentrate on. This control of the practice of meditation is often not helpful to you who are learning to meditate. If you are worried that you are not in the correct position, or do not have the correct environment surrounding you, i.e. incense, candles, soft music, neutral color, etc., or are not calling forth the correct mantra or image, you may become so frustrated that your mind will never leave the alpha state.

The ritual of candles and a certain place and sounds may work well for you. Or, you may be more comfortable just lying in bed in the morning, letting yourself go deeply into a meditative state. The use of meditation for healing and relaxing is a very personal thing, as is the use of any other tool. Because it is so personal, you need to develop the method of meditation which works best for you

How do I begin? You may lie down, sit, stand, walk or swim while you meditate. The idea is to find the position or action which feels most present or mindful to you. Those who are very active are often not comfortable sitting for long periods of time. You may feel much more calm and relaxed when slowly walking on a beach or a quiet path. Meditation works best when you find the most comfortable way to do it. Try them all, and your system will let you know what works.

Once you discover your way to comfortably calm yourself, decide on an object for your focus. This may be paying attention to your breath, using a word or phrase, calling forth a visual image, listening to a guiding tape or a piece of music, or gazing at something in nature. There are those who prefer to meditate with eyes slightly open, looking at the sky or a beautiful flower. When you discover that object to focus on, your job is to keep it in your mind for the duration of the meditation.

Is it easy? This said, although the concept, the philosophy of meditation sounds easy, the act is not. It may be the most difficult work you have ever done. The foolish mind wants to lead you in any direction except quiet. For example, you are calm and comfortable, you have decided on your focal object; you are ready. Immediately a number of irrelevant thoughts come tumbling into your head. The more you try to erase them, the stronger they become. Soon, you have completely forgotten your focal point and are worrying about what to cook for dinner, or why your energy is so low, or when you can bake a cake for your child's school Birthday party. The mind is a great diverter.

To change this, you may do a number of things. First, you may acknowledge each thought, as if it is a small child who needs your attention while you are on the phone. Actually say to each thought, "I hear you and I will take care of you in a few moments. Please wait over there", and designate a spot in your mind where thoughts may wait. Or, you may gently say to yourself, "I am returning to my focal point", and bring your attention back to it. Numbers work well for some when consistently diverted. Count slowly backwards from 20 to 1, breathing in and out with each number.

The idea is to keep at it without becoming discouraged. Everyone is innately able to meditate. If you focus on your personal object for only one minute, you have done it. Congratulate yourself and do it for one minute at a time until your mind allows you to go to two minutes. There is no magic number of minutes which is best for meditation. You may have read or heard that you need to meditate for at least 20 minutes to have it "work". Not so; it works if it is only for 20 seconds.

What if I have a problem relaxing? If you have a problem relaxing your body/mind, you may want to experiment with a couple of tricks. One, you can place your tongue on the roof of your mouth and take ten deep breaths. This position of the tongue may stop thoughts from tumbling into your brain. Or, breathing deeply, relax the tongue on the floor of the mouth, even allowing it to hang from the mouth slightly. The tongue often becomes tense when thoughts enter the brain; we even think with our tongues. You may also use a mask on your eyes, or cotton or a headset for your ears, or a "white noise" machine to block out external sounds. In other words, find what works and do it. When you are more comfortable with meditation, it will come easier for you.

Do you have any recommendations for success? Once you decide to meditate, you are already successful. However, I do recommend two things to deepen your internal journey. One, work to meditate at the same time each day. No, you do not need to have an empty stomach, or meditate first thing in the morning, or just before sunset. But since change is difficult, the body/mind responds more quickly to changes in schedule when they are the same each day. For example, you may want to meditate first thing in the morning. Wake, go to the bathroom, splash a bit of water on your face, then go back to bed, or sit in a chair, or whatever is most comfortable. Close your eyes, bring in your focal point, begin. Start with a minute, or two, or five; whichever feels best. Set a timer if you need to. After a few weeks, your body/mind will expect to meditate when you wake.

My second recommendation is to make sure you do not fall into a deep sleep while meditating. If lying down causes sleep, try propping yourself up; if you sleep while sitting, you may try this; as you breathe in, slightly raise one hand, and as you breathe out, lower it. This keeps the focus on the breath and the hand movement, usually keeping sleepiness at bay.

How will I know if it is working? You will know you are receiving benefits from meditation when you begin to experience certain signs. You will feel more focused, more in the present; you will deal with outer stress much more easily, since inner stress is diminished; you will feel a stronger sense of calmness, of content; others will be more comfortable around you, and you will be more comfortable with them. Your inner and outer balance will be deeper and stronger, your health will improve, life will be happier and more productive. This may all begin with one minute of focus today.

I strongly recommend this tool as one to include in your bag. If you are still distrustful of your ability to meditate, there an extensive list of books and other resources to help you discover your path to meditation in the back of this book. Often, those who feel they cannot meditate alone will utilize tapes, or meditate in a group or class. The group may choose to use the same focal point, perhaps a guiding tape, a piece of music or a candle, intensifying the energy in the meditation space. This may be a good place to begin. Or not. It is totally your choice, and your bag of tools.

A meditation for relaxation. Below is a short guided relaxation which may be taped and used to begin the process of meditation. When I began to meditate, I found it very hard to relax. I used an exercise like this one for a few weeks, then found I did not need it; my body/mind responded to two or three deep breaths.

If you decide to record this meditation, please stop for a period of two or three deep breaths each time you reach the "pause dots". This will ensure that you allow yourself enough time to take in each section and to relax fully. Good luck!

Close the eyes...breathe deeply into the belly....notice the path of the breath as it enters the body, and travels to the belly....notice the path of the breath as it leaves the body....breath in, breath out....begin to tune in to the small sounds around you....listen closely to each sound...just listen, noting any judgement or annoyance....now, tune in to the feeling of the outside of the body.... Bring your attention from the hair on the head, down to the toes on the feet.... notice which parts of the skin touch other things....clothing....the floor....a chair or bed....now, slowly bring the attention through the skin to the inside of the body....to the muscles, the bones, the organs....breathe deeply into the inner body....breathe in, breathe out....notice any emotion which may reside in the body....breathe into each emotion....breathe in, breathe out....no expectation, just noticing....notice that with each breath, the body/mind becomes more relaxed....deep breath in, deep breath out.... in, and out....more and more relaxed....into this relaxed body//mind, bring the symbol of focus chosen especially for you....notice it, and breathe deeply....in, and out....continue to relax and breathe deeply until you feel you need to return to your outer life...(Here, you may want to pause the recorder for as long as you feel comfortable, then resume)....bring your attention back slowly, gently......little by little....fully awake, fully aware, fully relaxed....

CASE STUDIES

INTRODUCTION

In the following pages, you will read the brief health histories of five clients. These histories are compounded from the many clients who have come to me for counseling and inner balance work. The names of the clients have been changed, as well as much of the personal information. The issues they presented remain intact, as do the contracts for deeper balance agreed upon by them

Clare: "I don't know what I want"

"I don't know where to go from here" Clare half-whispers in a small tense voice as she curls up on the couch, holding a pillow against her to protect her middle. "I've been to lots of therapists, no one can help me." I question her concerning past counseling experience, and discover that she has seen a Behaviorist who had criticized her for not following the rules, a young woman Psychologist who had offered advice, but had not really listened to her, and an older man who after hearing her story and seeing her for two sessions, suggested that she probably should see a woman. She then contacted me.

"What do you want from me?" I ask. Clare begins to sob. "No one ever asked me that," she says when she is able to speak clearly. "I don't know what I want anymore, from you or from myself."

Clare is in her middle forties. She is married and has two teenage sons. She is pale, listless, very thin. She cries a lot over nothing, she says. She has low blood pressure, chronic lower back pain, migraine headaches which occur two to three times monthly, and has just been diagnosed with Fibromyalgia, which causes pain in her back, legs and shoulders, especially at night. She eats very little, takes three medications daily and drinks a glass of wine before her evening meal. She has plenty of money, she states, but she does not see her husband very much. He owns a large plumbing company and works long hours, burying himself in his job. Her sons are never home, because they are involved in sport, school and their friends. She has few close friends, does not belong to an organized religion, and her family lives in another state.

Clare's physician has adjusted her medication for depression three times. She also takes pain medications for her back and Fibromyalgia, and a sleeping pill every other night. She states that she sometimes takes a multi-vitamin, although not every day. She tries to walk a mile three times weekly, and sometimes watches a video for stretching exercise. She is aware that she needs to eat a more balanced diet, but food does not interest her. Her diet often consists of a few pieces of fruit, several cups of tea, crackers with cheese or peanut butter. She is fond of sweets, so takes bites of cake or ice cream or cookies throughout the day. She eats a balanced meal of chicken, vegetables and rice perhaps twice weekly, to assuage the guilt of eating too much sugar.

She does not discuss her problems with friends or family. Her basic emotion is weeping. She does not feel anger, or joy. She has considered suicide, but would not carry through with it because it would devastate her boys. She often wants to go to sleep and never wake up.

Following explanation of the services I offer, we make a contract for six weeks of nutritional and psychotherapeutic counseling. We agree to discuss other alternatives for energy balance if she feels better after this time. Clare agrees to follow a few contracted dietary changes, take supplements, and to attend all of her appointments.

Dietary changes for Clare involve eating one balanced meal each day, choosing foods containing less sweetness and more oil and protein, taking a regular supplement twice daily, and continuation of her regular meds. Following six weeks of counseling and the changes in diet, Clare is smiling a bit more, and sleeping better. Her weeping has diminished some, and she has only experienced one migraine in six weeks.

Since she feels more in charge of her life, Clare is eager to contract for other alternative services. I explain my services again, and also share information about acupuncture and herbal medicine, along with those providers whom I would recommend in her area. Clare contracts for a visit with an Oriental Medicine Physician, who provides both acupuncture and Herbal medicine. She wishes only to have an evaluation, and not to commit to treatment at this time. She will contract for six more weeks of counseling, however, amd will do some simple deep breathing exercises each morning on awakening. Another suggestion she feels she may follow is to spend a few hours each week helping someone.

Six weeks later, Clare states that she has received three acupuncture treatments, and is taking Chinese herbs daily. (She says the needles don't hurt but she does not like them; she closes her eyes and takes deep breaths during treatment). Her appetite has improved and she enjoys her food more; she has been free of headaches for over four weeks; she is sleeping well; she has not wept in three weeks. She has given up most sweet foods, and the Fibromyalgia is somewhat improved. She has joined a club with a pool, and is swimming twice a week. Her blood pressure has improved. She has decided to volunteer at a local library, reading to children two hours weekly.

"I feel like I want to live, finally," she states with a small smile.

In the following year, Clare returned for four single counseling sessions. She continued to receive acupuncture once monthly and herbal medicine daily, to improve her diet and to do the Breathwork 10 minutes daily. When I heard from her last, she was medication free, and was preparing for her older son's wedding.

Comments:

Clare was in her forties, and although in emotional distress and dealing with some immune system depletion, had not yet suffered deep systemic imbalance. One year of alternative treatment and counseling made a huge difference in her life. She was committed to improving her health, and definitely on her way to consistent inner balance, and a happier last half of her life.

Please realize that Clare did not feel better because the acupuncturist stuck needles in her, or because I guided her through Psychosynthesis counseling, or because she was eating a better diet. She felt better because she utilized her inner will in her quest to be more healthy. No amount of counseling or alternative balancing work will make you better if you do not participate fully. You are the one who is ill; you are the only one who can make yourself better. Change is difficult for all of us; when you decide to change, it is very important to choose someone who will work with you, not against you. Change only happens at your pace, not that of someone else. The rules for change need to be yours, or you will not follow them. The inner will is very strong concerning this. It knows, even when the mind does not, that what is being offered is either what has come before, and will harm, or what feels totally right, and will heal. Counseling is the most important tool for accessing the inner will. Therefore, the counselor must be fully aware of this.

At no time was Clare advised to stop taking medications. Because her body was feeling lighter, more healthy and her depression was waning, she opted, with her doctor's advice, to lessen the meds, then finally to stop them. The balanced system does not need synthetic drugs. As the body becomes more healthy, the need for them often diminishes, then disappears altogether. Herbal medicine and supplements may be needed for years following the stoppage of drugs, but keep in mind that these substances are not synthetic, and are accepted quite well by the body.

Geoff: "It began with a macrobiotic diet"

Geoff is 38 years old, 5 feet 8 inches tall, and weighs 93 pounds when he first comes to me for a consultation. He is extremely thin, has gaunt pale cheeks, sunken eye-sockets, a sweetish odor and is covered with a downy "fur" on his face, chest and back. He has thick black hair and blue eyes. He wears a number of layers of clothing, stating that he is always chilled. Geoff is married and has one daughter. He works at a middle-management position in a large organization. He is consistently fatigued, has low blood pressure, sleeps poorly and his back, knees, shoulders and neck ache when he sits for long periods of time. He severely limits his daily food intake, often eating only 600 calories, and runs or jogs 5-6 miles each evening. He takes no medicines or supplements. Geoff has been medically and psychiatrically diagnosed with anorexia nervosa.

"Why are you here?" I ask. Geoff tells me he began to eat a macrobiotic diet three years before, and found himself limiting his food intake more each week, until he was eating only brown rice two times daily. He is not following a macro-biotic regimen presently, but he is unable to eat more than a little food each day, because it makes him feel bloated and heavy. For the past three months Geoff has experienced a need to "run off" his larger evening meal. He has been told that if he continues with his present regimen of eating too little and exercising too rigor-ously, he is at grave risk of dying from a heart attack. He does not see himself as thin, but he believes those who have advised him. Geoff is afraid of death, and wishes to investigate alternative methods to wellness, and to be able to eat enough to maintain a healthy weight.

I state that although I am a Nutritionist, I am not willing to contract nutrition work with those with severe eating disorders. He must find a nutritionist as part of his therapy, and must see a physician who will work with the three of us while we discover his path to balance. We agree to six weekly counseling sessions and deep Breathwork for 10 minutes daily. Geoff is also willing to take a multiple vitamin and mineral and a bit of zinc daily, and to run 4 miles daily rather than 6. He is not willing to add calories to his diet or to see a Nutritionist at this time. He will inform his doctor that we are meeting. He agrees not to discuss his nutri-tional needs with me.

Following six weeks of counseling, Geoff has not gained weight, and admits that he has not fulfilled his agreement to run less. He is taking vitamins and doing deep breathing, and he is sleeping somewhat better. He fears if he eats he will suffer cramps in his gut, since this has happened in the past.

At this point, I state that I am not willing to contract for more counseling with Geoff until he has kept an appointment with a Nutritionist, and brings me a program that they agree on for steady weight gain. Geoff chooses to terminate counseling, asking me if he may return if he changes his mind. I agree to see him if he maintains his present weight, or gains weight.

Two months later, Geoff calls me and informs me that he has located a Nutritionist he is willing to work with, and wishes to return for counseling. He states that he continues to take his supplements, and has not stopped his Breathwork. Geoff has not lost weight, so I agree to see him for further counseling.

Geoff and I agree to weekly counseling on a month-to-month basis for an undetermined amount of time. He sees a Nutritionist once monthly, and monitors his progress with his physician quarterly. After 4 months of counseling, Geoff agrees to see an Acupuncturist for evaluation, and to take herbs if they are recommended. Herbal therapy and regular acupuncture appointments are begun soon after, and Geoff attends all appointments.

Geoff and his Nutritionist agreed on a weight of 125 pounds, since Geoff fears becoming too fat and uncomfortable. Geoff and I agree on a modified exercise regimen, with Geoff jogging three times weekly for two miles, and doing resistance training for 20 minutes three times weekly to build his muscle tone.

After 14 months, Geoff has gained 20 pounds. His color has improved, his blood pressure is rising, his electrolytes are balanced, he sleeps more soundly. The furry matter on his skin is gone, as is the sweet odor. Still very thin and pale, he is 12 pounds under his goal of 125. We agree to continue meeting monthly. Geoff agrees to see the Nutritionist quarterly, and to check with his physician twice yearly. We discuss further alternative treatments, and Geoff agrees to trade a weekly Yoga session for one 2-mile run.

Geoff and I work together for more than 4 years. At our last meeting, he weighs 123 pounds and states that it is difficult for him to maintain that high weight, but he is doing it because he knows that his wife and daughter need him and he will die if he allows himself to slip back into his anorexic habits. He states that his stomach often bothers him, especially when he eats too much, and that he still experiences bouts of fatigue. He also states that he feels more content, and that he almost always sleeps well. He informs me that he is fully aware that if he had not utilized alternative treatments, he is certain he would not be here now.

Comments:

Anorexia nervosa is an insidious disease. When Geoff and I first met, he was in the last stage of depletion from the disease. The furry appearance of the skin and the unusual odor signify a grave inner imbalance in minerals needed to help the body work properly, called electrolytes. The one thing he was not experiencing was a psychosis. Often, those in last stages are thoroughly convinced that they are doing the right thing, and that they are fat and will never be able to eat small enough amounts to become truly thin. They see themselves in mirrors as fat. This is called distorted body image. No amount of counseling or cajoling will change their minds. A large percentage of those in this stage die, usually because the heart cannot continue with so little nutritional support.

I choose not to work with nutrition when a client presents with a severe eating disorder, since the client often is very knowledgeable regarding nutrition, and may use this knowledge to control his sessions away from dealing with deeper issues. Eating disorders are symptoms of deeper imbalance, and the reasons for this need to be addressed if the client is to regain his health.

Geoff often felt out of control in every area of his life. Food intake was one thing he could control. We needed to find a balance between his need to control treatment, and my comfort, since I might have been liable if Geoff died while we worked together. We agreed together that I needed this protection. This was accomplished by my assurance that Geoff received nutritional and medical supervision on a consistent basis outside counseling. Once that was established, we could work with Geoff's inner will, within our sessions.

Geoff made very good progress for a person in his depleted condition. Anorexics often do not agree to maintain a healthy body weight, and continue to find occasions to starve themselves, to maintain what they feel is control. Geoff felt that acupuncture and herbal treatments contributed greatly to his ability to maintain inner health and balance. Our hope is that he will continue to utilize these treatments to grow toward deeper contentment and balance.

Miriam: "I do what everyone tells me; why do I still feel lousy?"

"I don't know why I'm here, really. I guess it's because I'm sick of being sick. I have seen so many doctors. They don't help me, they just give me more pills, or suggest more operations. I need to feel better." Miriam is 56 years old, and has not felt healthy most of her adult life. She has had rheumatoid arthritis since her mid twenties, her blood pressure and cholesterol levels are in the high normal range, she has a compromised digestive system due to ingestion of medication, and she suffers from frequent bladder and kidney infections. She is thin and pale, her hair is colorless and wispy, her skin is dry with a yellowish caste. She moves slowly and with pain, and her wrists and knees appear swollen. She eats and sleeps poorly, and is often extremely fatigued. She has had both knees and one hip replaced due to joint deterioration. Presently she is experiencing pain in both wrists, elbows and shoulders, and in her lower back.

Miriam has been married for 35 years, and has two children and three grand-children. She shares that her husband and son did not want her to see me, fearful that "you might do something weird to me." She smiles wryly as she tells me this, stating that nothing could be as weird as some of the things that have already been done to her, referring to the joint replacements. Miriam feels that if she had known how to prevent these procedures, she would have.

When arthritis was diagnosed, Miriam decided she would follow her physicians' advice, because she believed they must know best. She placed herself into their hands, hoping with each new treatment for complete remission of the disease. The arthritis did abate somewhat following two of the treatments, only to return months later. Miriam now has severe skeletal damage in many of her joints. The disease has not affected her organs to date. The problems with her kidneys and stomach stem from ingestion of medication.

Miriam eats poorly, preferring soft foods which she feels are easier to digest, tea and a glass of wine two or three times weekly. She takes no supplements, and eats few fresh fruits or vegetables. She drinks very little water. Miriam is presently taking medications to reduce inflammation, to help her digest her food, to aid in sleep and to normalize her blood pressure. She has recently terminated a course of antibiotics for a kidney infection.

Miriam is unable to work, gets out very little, and has a poor relationship with her husband and her son. She does not feel much love for either, stating that they pity her, and she does not like to be pitied. She says that she has remained in her marriage because her husband agreed to care for her. She fears that if he does not approve of her care, he will not pay for it. He has agreed to a limited amount of sessions with me, but he needs to see some progress to allow her to continue. Her daughter is very supportive of her seeking any care which might help her mother to improve.

I explain in detail those alternative procedures I am familiar with, and recommend that Miriam become more familiar with them before committing herself to what will probably be long-term alternative care. I also recommend that along with nutritional and spiritual counseling, she have a consultation with an Acupuncturist who is able to provide her with Traditional Chinese herbal Medicine as he treats her, and to see a doctor of Chiropractic to see if her skeletal damage can be improved. I also suggest Meditation and Breathwork, which involve no financial burden, and gentle massage once monthly to relax tight muscles.

Miriam is anxious to begin all of this work at once. I suggest she and her husband spend a month reading about the various procedures, and that at the end of that time she return with her husband to discuss a treatment plan. Miriam is anxious about informing her husband that he needs to see me. I share with her that without his co-operation, she may not be able to receive enough care to achieve her goal of improved inner balance and more robust health.

Miriam returns in a month with her husband Thomas. They have read the pamphlets and books I recommended, and are ready to discuss her treatment. Thomas is still skeptical of alternative treatment. I inform him that it is indeed different from medical treatment, in that most forms take permanent healing of the entire system into consideration, rather than treating symptoms. I also inform them that results may take longer than they anticipate. Miriam is used to treatment with drugs, the effects of which may occur within days or weeks. I tell Miriam and Thomas that her treatment may take years, since the body needs to reverse damage that has taken so many years to accumulate.

This disturbs Miriam, who had hoped that if she followed all of the procedures, she would see results in a short period of time. She is so upset by this news that she decides not to enter into a contract at this time, but to take a month more to consider what I have said.

Miriam calls me three weeks later, and tells me that she and Thomas have agreed that she needs to do something other than follow the regime she has used for over thirty years. She hopes for a better quality of life than she has experienced, and fears that medications alone will not supply this for her. We meet again, and formulate a plan for intensive alternative treatment.

Rather than consider the usual six-week contract, we agree to six months of treatment. Miriam will remain with her program for the duration, even though she realizes that immmediate results may not be forthcoming. Thomas reluctantly agrees to support this plan. Miriam will continue to take her prescribed medications during this time. Her doctor has been informed of her decision, and although not knowledgeable of some of the procedures, wishes her well on her journey to wellness.

Miriam's six-month program consists of weekly counseling sessions for nutrition and spiritual wellness, evaluation for acupuncture and herbal medicine treatments as prescribed by a doctor of TCM, Breathwork and Meditation for twenty minutes each day, Massage once each month, and Chiropractic care when necessary. Miriam locates those practitioners with whom she feels comfortable within two months, and is able to attend most of her appointments.

"This is a lot of work," she declares when she, Thomas and I met for her six-month evaluation. "Worth every minute and penny of it, though," Thomas counters with a broad smile. "Just look at her." Miriam looks more relaxed, smiles more, her hair has taken on a sheen and seems thicker, and her skin has lost much of its yellow color. She is sleeping better and eats more regular meals. She still experiences pain, but it seems more bearable. She has been able to attend two social functions in the past month, and she and Thomas are going to dinner together one night a week, something he declares they have not done in years.

Miriam is looking forward to being able to play bridge weekly again. She also wishes to travel in two months to see her grandson celebrate his bar mitzvah 2000 miles away. "I plan to dance at my daughter's wedding some day, too," she says coyly, "if she ever decides to settle down." Miriam continues to take all medications except sleeping pills, which she feels she does not need.

Miriam has a long journey to wellness ahead of her. We continue counseling sessions once a month for another six months, then she comes when she feels the need. She continues intensive acupuncture treatment for a year, also, then is able to limit treatment to once monthly. She is not able to see the massage therapist each month, but plans to have massage three or four times yearly. She sees a Chiropractor monthly. She realizes she will need to continue to balance her diet for a lifetime with herbs and other food supplements, which will be adjusted on a regular basis. She continues to eat carefully, avoiding dairy products, sugar, alcohol, caffeine and fatty meat, and eating more raw foods and complex grains, nuts and seeds as her digestion improves.

I move while Miriam is still working with me periodically. We meet to evaluate her progress before we terminate our time together. It has been over seven years since Miriam and Thomas first committed themselves to her path to greater balance and wellness. Miriam is now relatively pain-free, needing only small doses of Ibuprophen at times to control inflammation; she takes prescribed medication only for her digestive system, which has suffered severe damage and needs regular care to assure that she remains free of acid reflux. She receives acupuncture 6-8 times yearly, and massage and Chiropractic treatments when needed; she continues to practice breathwork and meditation on a regular basis., and is swimming three times weekly and taking a therapeutic yoga class.

Miriam has not experienced bladder or kidney infections for over four years. She sleeps well and stretches for 10 minutes on waking. Miriam's skeletal damage still exists, but because she is more relaxed and her muscles are consistently stretched, she experiences much greater range of motion.

Miriam and her husband are now getting along well; she stated that he has gained respect for her work, and no longer pities her. Her son has grudgingly accepted her progress, and they are working on a more peaceful relationship. Her 37 year old daughter married the year before, and Miriam delights in telling me that she danced at her wedding.

Comments:

Miriam needed a lot of courage to begin to walk her path to wellness. She had been very ill for many years, and she was fully aware that it would take a long time before she felt really healthy. Her arthritic condition did not respond well to even the most sophisticated new medicines recommended by her rheumatologist. She learned that much of her illness was due to her giving herself over to others, not just physicians but many people in her life. When she began to take charge of her own process toward wellness, she began to recover more quickly.

Miriam's path is not for everyone. It can be very time-consuming and financially burdening. Because Miriam and her husband committed themselves to her work, and because she could financially afford to receive multiple treatments at once, her work progressed quite quickly.

Lack of finances to jump into lots of alternative treatment does not mean that you cannot become well, no matter what your financial state or time commitment may be. If you have been chronically ill for years, you may still find a program which will allow you to evolve into wellness. You may want to locate a holistic counselor in your area, and develop a plan together which will allow you to progress toward balance at your own pace. Know that is is far better to take one small step forward than to remain stuck in the same place, or continue sliding into more severe and chronic illness.

It is important to seek care that is supportive. I cannot say this often enough. Physicians often have no training in or knowledge of alternative practices, but you may find a physician who supports you on your path, as Miriam did. I once left the long-time care of my physician when he pooh-poohed my alternative treatments as "poppycock", and attributed my progress toward health to my positive marriage.

Positive relationships are very important in the larger scheme of things, but no healing process can work with just one tool. All the love in the world could not change my diet, or balance my organs, or supply me with the proper herbs, foods and supplements. A complete, personal bag of tools and the commitment to use them are needed for balance and robust health.

Barry: "I don't really feel sick, just tired all the time"

When I first meet with Barry, he is 48 years old. He has been working since he was 19, having completed his college education at an early age. He is now an upper-level administrator, and works almost 60 hours a week. He is divorced from a 20 year marriage, and when not working he is eating or sleeping. Barry is tall and of a normal weight, very pale, quiet, slow-moving and lacking energy. His diet consists of pastries or donuts for breakfast, fast food from the cafeteria at work or restaurants, or processed foods in the form of frozen dinners. He has one or two mixed drinks each night, more on the weekends. His voice is thin and feathery, he is fatigued, and his breath is shallow and thready. His legs, neck and shoulders often ache, and he has an unusual blood pressure which averages 105/100. His triglycerides are unusually high, but his cholesterol readings are within normal range. Barry takes two tablets of Ibuprophen when needed for his aches, but takes no prescribed medication. He does, however, rely on one or two antacids following each meal.

Barry states that he is not content with his life, and although he is not often ill, he is often fatigued. He is dating a woman whom he did not love, but he has not broken off the relationship because he fears hurting her. He is in grave financial difficulty, having agreed to allot most of his income to his ex-wife and his teenaged son. He states that he is usually not aware of his feelings, but that lately he finds that when he rubs his achey legs, he will sometimes cry.

Barry saw a male counselor for four sessions shortly before he was divorced. He states that his decision to divorce came while in counseling. He left his marriage because he did not love his wife, but felt guilty because he loved another woman at the time of the divorce. When she left him shortly after the divorce, he became lonely. He does not wish to return to his ex-wife, but he wants a partner.

Barry contracts for six weeks of nutritional and emotional counseling. He states that he is not prepared to contract for other work at that time. He will agree to change his diet to some degree, and to take supplements if he is able take them first thing in the morning.

Following the six weeks of counseling and changes in diet tailored to lower triglycerides and to introduce fewer processed foods, less trans-fat and dairy products and more lean protein, Barry announces that his consumption of antacids is reduced by half, he is feeling somewhat more energetic and his legs do not ache as much. He feels ready to discuss options for speeding up his healing. We discuss including regular breathing exercises to deepen his shallow breath and increase energy movement, massage once a month to relieve his aches, and acupuncture for deeper inner balance and faster resolution of his fatigue. While discussing an exercise program, Barry reveals that he loved to play golf in his youth, and gave it up because his ex-wife did not approve of his taking time off from his family on the weekends.

Barry contracts to find a massage therapist, to seek an Acupuncturist for evaluation, to commit to breathwork 10 minutes daily and to receive six further weeks of counseling. "If it'll resolve things fast, I'm in", he states.

During our second contract, Barry begins six sessions of acupuncture. He experiences one massage, and shares that he slept deeply and well following it, and plans to return each month. Barry also participated in two guided sessions of Psychosynthesis counseling, and played a round of golf with rented clubs. He continues to follow his adjusted diet, and has limited his intake of alcohol to one drink per night during the week and two on the weekends. He terminated the relationship with the woman he had been dating, and had a date the following weekend with a woman he connected with on the golf course. "I'm obviously feeling better, as you can see," he comments.

Barry receives much benefit from his acupuncture sessions, and is able to reduce his counseling sessions to one each month. He receives monthly massage, practices deep breathing 10 minutes daily, and plays golf whenever his busy schedule allows. Four months after beginning healing work, Barry's triglycerides are within normal range. Eight months after beginning his work, Barry' s job transfers him to another state. At our last meeting, he states that he feels better than he has in years, and definitely plans to continue with his new routine.

Comments:

Although Barry was aggressive at his job, he tended toward passivity in relationships. He also displayed resistance to many changes at one time. When allowed to set his own pace and name his terms for change, Barry firmly stuck to his schedule, and was able to see great changes in a short period of time.

It is very important that the providers who work with you as you grow are fully invested in helping you to become a unique individual who will grow in your own time and at your own pace. Although I might assume that Barry would benefit greatly from Psychosynthesis counseling, his need to control his healing process must come before my need to speed it up with work I assumed would be right for him. It was necessary for me to place my ego needs aside to help Barry gain control of and deepen the balance in his life.

When seeking a provider, be certain that you do not feel pushed into change before you are prepared to accept it. Change that is achieved in this manner often is not permanent. You may feel as if you have changed, but if you find yourself slipping back, it may be due to the fact that the inner will was not ready, and felt pushed. It will then revert back to former patterns, and retreat into what feels more comfortable, more right. What really happens is that this is the only control that the will knows, and so it employs it. New controls occur only when the inner will has complete permission to change, both from outside and from within, and sets its adjusted rules and boundaries according to your unique system.

Angela: "I've been fat forever. I hate it."

Angela sits on the small couch, her fingers laced across her stomach. Her legs stick straight out before her. She is just under 5 feet tall, and weighs 234 pounds. She is 33 years old, married and has a 9 year old son. Angela has smooth pink skin, naturally curly dark hair, and is carefully made up. Her smile reveals even white teeth and a dimple in one cheek.

Angela is morbidly obese, meaning that she is at least 100 pounds heavier than the highest healthy weight for her size and structure. She grew up in a fat family. Her mother, father, two brothers and one sister are all considerably overweight. Angela was a fat child and has matured into a fatter adult. She has never been thin. Her movement has become impaired in the past two years. It is more difficult for her to climb stairs, due to pain in her ankles and knees. Her back bothered her during pregnancy, so she spent most of her last trimester in a chair. Her son was a normal birth, but Angela lost only 10 of the 52 pounds she gained during pregnancy. Angela's husband has a big appetite but is normal weight, and loves her at her size, she states. She has dieted half-heartedly for years, only to put on more than the 15 to 20 pounds she has lost. Her husband and family do not actively support weight loss, stating that she is fine the way she is.

At this time, Angela is often tired and experiences pain in her back, knees, neck and shoulders. Her digestion is not good and she is not sleeping well. The last time she saw a doctor, she was told that her glucose count was 134, bordering on high, and that she needed to be aware of her intake of sweets or she may develop Type 2 diabetes. Her diet consists of no breakfast, large meals at midday and in the evening, sweet and crunchy snacks between meals and before bedtime. She drinks lots of sweet fruit juices, but no caffeine or alcohol. She often eats at fast-food restaurants, and prepares meals with packaged foods.

Angela spends most of her social time with her family, talking around the table while eating large meals, and sitting in front of TV. She loves to read, and takes her son to the library or to a bookstore on a regular basis. Her son is a normal weight, but she is worried that she is passing her poor eating habits to him, and that he will be fat when he is older. The only time Angela has exercise is when she cleans house or walks in the mall.

Angela is aware that she "eats her emotions", meaning when she feels lonely, sad or angry, she reaches for something sweet. Food is her tranquillizer, she states. She learned this from watching an Oprah Winfrey program, and was appalled when she realized this applied to her. She cannot understand why her life remains the same, even after she has discovered why she eats. Angela takes a prescribed medication to prevent acid buildup in her stomach, and a sleeping pill two or three times weekly. She also takes 2-4 tablets of Ibuprophen daily for her aches. She takes no supplements.

Angela contracts for six weeks of counseling and some minor diet changes. Although she wishes to be thinner, she is not willing at this time to follow a strict diet. This feels too stressful for her. We discuss what she is willing to do, and she decides to begin a program of deep breathing 10 minutes daily. She also agrees to walk 3-5 minutes after her evening meal. We decide not to weigh her until she has completed her first contract.

Six weeks later, following small changes in diet, a regimen of deep breathing and a very short daily walk, Angela has lost 8 pounds. She is very surprised. She does not think she worked very hard to achieve that, she states. She has agreed to begin eating breakfast, which consists of a glass of comfortably hot water with the juice of one-half lemon in it, one piece of whole grain toast with peanut butter and a cup of herb tea with lemon and a little honey. She also agrees to drink her juices made with half water and half juice, and not to limit, but to observe herself eating between meal snacks. She does not agree to limit or measure any of her meals, but discovers that she is also observing herself eat at meals, and will sometimes stop before she finishes them, feeling that she does not really want that much food. She apologises for not fulfilling her walking contract each day, since her ankles hurt on three occasions and she does not want to walk. She says she sat in a chair in front of TV those three days and pumped her legs for three minutes. When asked why, she says she promised to fill the contract, and she really wanted to do something.

"What's my next step?" She asks eagerly. I ask her where she is willing to go from here. Angela decides on six more weeks of counseling, and is willing to make a few more small changes in her diet. She agrees to take supplements once daily, and to give up between meal snacks during the day, stating that she is not ready to give up her nighttime snacks. She will continue with her Breathwork, and with her walking contract, but wishes to change it so if she is sore, she can substitute leg-pumping instead.

Following her second six-week contract, Angela has lost 16 pounds. Her back feels somewhat better, and she is able to fulfill her walking contract on all but two nights and to progress from three minutes to five each night. She states that her family is leaving her alone because she informed them that she wanted to be in charge of herself, and she didn't like herself so fat. She told them she would not listen to them unless they gave her positive moral support. Her husband agreed, as did her mother. Her brothers and father are not commenting. Angela is taking fewer sleeping pills, and she is taking half of her former dosage of stomach medication. Her glucose levels have been normal for three weeks.

Angela continues to come for counseling once a month for one year. At the end of this time, she has given up between meal snacks, is drinking much less juice and more water, has added salads and some whole foods to her diet, and limits her sweets to special treats. She now walks 10 minutes after her evening meals, walks the length of the mall twice a month with her mother, and takes a weekly yoga class for larger women. She continues her deep breathing daily. Angela has lost 47 pounds. She weighs herself once a month. Angela now knows how she feels emotionally most of the time, and is able to express her feelings in a journal or to me instead of reaching for food to mask them.

Comments:

Angela's eating patterns were very deeply and culturally ingrained, and were an integral part of the person she had become. Rather than approaching weight loss with bahavior modification, we decided not to deal with the issue of weight loss at all, but to approach Angela's balancing work with steps to better health. Thin is not always better, when overweight bodies are the rule in families. Many things need to be considered, not the least of which is acceptance and love from those you live with and respect. When we are deprived of this love and acceptance, we can become more ill.

Not many will argue with improvement in health, however, so we contracted to take this approach. Because this appealed so much to Angela, it worked well. She was working to become more healthy and balanced, not to be thin. She could easily defend and find both inner and outer support for this approach. Her mother actually began to follow her program toward the end of the year, when she saw that her daughter was much healthier and happier, and she realized that Angela had not felt deprived during this process.

Angela may need counseling support for some time, on a part-time basis. She is not willing to receive acupuncture for deeper balance, or to take herbal medicine, although she has become aware that these approaches may assure faster healing, or deeper changes in cellular balance. Counseling, exercise and breathwork will assist in her work, but may take longer. Meanwhile, Angela continues to improve in health and balance.

RECOMMENDED READING

Counseling

Bourne, Edmund J., and Lorna Garano, *Coping with Anxiety: 10 Simple Ways to Relieve Anxiety, Fear, and Worry*, New Harbinger Publications, 2003.

Bourne, Edmund J., *Beyond Anxiety and Phobia: A Step-by-Step Guide to Lifetime Recovery*, New Harbinger Publications, 2001.

Bourne, Edmund J., *The Anxiety and Phobia Workbook*, New Harbinger Publications, 3rd Ed., 2000.

Breggin, Peter R., M.D., *The Anti-Depressant Fact Book: What Your Doctor Won't Tell You About Prozac, Zoloft, Paxil, Celexa, and Luvox*, Perseus Publishing, 2001.

Breggin, Peter R., M.D., *Toxic Psychiatry: Why Therapy, Empathy and Love Must Replace the Drugs, Electroshock, and Biochemical Theories of the "New Psychiatry,"* St. Martin's Griffin, 1994.

Glasser, William, *Counseling with Choice Theory*, Perennial, 2001.

Hardin, Jerry D., and Dianne C. Sloan, *Getting Ready for Marriage Workbook: How to Really Get to Know the Person You're Going to Marry*, Nelson Books, 1992.

Littrell, John M., *Brief Counseling in Action*, W.W. Norton & Co., 1998.

Louden, Jennifer, *The Woman's Comfort Book: A Self-Nurturing Guide for Restoring Balance in Your Life*, HarperSanFrancisco, 1992.

Louden, Jennifer, *The Woman's Retreat Book: A Guide to Restoring, Rediscovering, and Reawakening Your True Self in a Moment, an Hour, a Day, or a Weekend*, HarperSanFrancisco, 1997.

McGraw, Jay, *Life Strategies for Teens*, Fireside, 2000.

McGraw, Phil, *Relationship Rescue: A Seven Step Strategy for Reconnecting with Your Partner*, Hyperion, 2001.

McGraw, Phil, *The Relationship Rescue Workbook*, Hyperion, 2000.

Palmer, Pat, and Melissa Alberti Froehner, *Teen Esteem: A Self-Direction Manual for Young Adults*, 2nd. Ed., Little Imp, 2000.

Rinpoche, Sogyal, *The Tibetan Book of Living and Dying: The Spiritual Classic and International Bestseller, Revised and Updated Edition,* HarperSanFrancisco, 1994.

Wilson, Sandra D., *Released from Shame: Recovery for Adult Children of Dysfunctional Families,* InterVarsity Press, 1991.

Nutrition

Bauer, Joy, *The Complete Idiot's Guide to Total Nutrition, 3rd Edition*, Alpha Books, 2002.

Beale, Lucy, and Sandy Couvillon, *The Complete Idiot's Guide to Weight Loss*, Alpha Books, 2002.

Beck, Martha, *The Joy Diet: 10 Daily Practices for a Happier Life*, Crown, 2003.

Brody, Jane E., *Jane Brody's Nutrition Book: A Lifetime Guide to Good Eating for Better Health and Weight Control*, W.W. Norton & Co., 1984.

Buono, Anthony, *The Race Against Junk Food (Adventures in Good Nutrition)*, HCom, 1997.

Campbell, T. Colin, *The China Study: The Most Comprehensive Study of Nutrition Ever Conducted and the Startling Implications for Diet, Weight Loss and Long-Term Health*, Benbella Books, 2005.

Coulter, H. David, *Anatomy of Hatha Yoga: A Manual for Students, Teachers, and Practitioners*, Body and Breath, 2001.

Ely, Leanne, *Healthy Foods: An Irreverent Guide to Understanding Nutrition and Feeding Your Family Well*, Champion Press, 2001.

Farhi, Donna, *Yoga Mind, Body & Spirit: A Return to Wholeness*, Owl Books, 2000.

Gottlieb, Jeff and Martha, *Spriggles Motivational Books for Children: Health and Nutrition*, Mountain Watch Press, 2001.

Leedy, Loreen, *The Edible Pyramid: Good Eating Every Day*, Holiday House, 1996.

MacWilliam, Lyle, *Comparative Guide to Nutritional Supplements*, Northern Dimensions Publishing, 2003.

Phillips, Bill, *Eating for Life: Your Guide to Great Health, Fat Loss, and Increased Energy!*, High Point Media, 2003.

Pitchford, Paul, *Healing with Whole Foods: Asian Traditions and Modern Nutrition,* 3ʳᵈ Edition, North Atlantic Books, 2002.

Rinzler, Carol Ann, *Nutrition for Dummies,* For Dummies, 3ʳᵈ Ed., 2003.

Saltman, Paul, Joel Gurin, and Ira Mothner, *The University of California San Diego Nutrition Book,* Little, Brown, 1993.

Schiffman, Erich, *Yoga: The Spirit and Practice of Moving Into Stillness,* Pocket, 1996.

Sears, William, M.D., Martha Sears, and Christie Kelly, *Eat Healthy, Feel Great,* Little, Brown, 2002.

Strand, Ray, M.D., *What Your Doctor Doesn't Know About Nutritional Medicine May Be Killing You,* Nelson Books, 2002.

Tenney, Louise, *Today's Herbal Health for Children: A Comprehensive Guide to Understanding Nutrition and Herbal Medicine for Children,* Woodland Publishing, 1996.

Willett, Walter C., M.D., *Eat, Drink, and Be Healthy: The Harvard Medical School Guide to Healthy Eating,* Free Press, 2002.

Acupuncture

Dolowich, Gary, M.D., *Archetypal Acupuncture: Healing with the Five Elements,* Jade Mountain, 2004.

Ellis, Andrew, et al., *Fundamentals of Chinese Acupuncture,* Rev. Ed., Paradigm Publications, 1991.

Johns, Robert, *The Art of Acupuncture Techniques,* North Atlantic Books, 1996.

Kaptchuk, Ted J., *The Web that Has No Weaver: Understanding Chinese Medicine,* McGraw-Hill, 2000.

Kenyon, Julian, M.D., *Acupressure Techniques: A Self-Help Guide,* Healing Arts Press, 1996.

Kidson, Dr. Ruth, *Acupuncture for Everyone: What It Is, Why It Works, and How It Can Help You,* Healing Arts Press, 2001.

Rothfeld, Glenn S., and Suzanne LeVert, *Natural Medicine for Arthritis: The Best Alternative Methods for Relieving Pain and Stiffness: From Food & Herbs to Acupuncture & Homeopathy,* Rodale Press, 1996.

Sollars, David, *Complete Idiot's Guide to Acupuncture and Acupressure,* Alpha Books, 2000.

Stux, Gabriel, et al., *Basics of Acupuncture,* 5th Rev. Ed., Springer-Verlag, 2003.

Homeopathy

Castro, Miranda, *The Complete Homeopathy Handbook: Safe and Effective Ways to Treat Fevers, Coughs, Colds, and Sore Throats, Childhood Ailments, Food Poisoning, Flu, and a Wide Range of Everyday Complaints,* St. Martin's Griffin, 1991.

Chappell, Peter, *Emotional Healing with Homeopathy: Treating the Effects of Trauma,* North Atlantic Books, 2003.

Cummings, Stephen, M.D., and Dana Ullman, *Everybody's Guide to Homeopathic Medicines: Safe and Effective Remedies for You and Your Family,* 3rd Rev. Ed., Jeremy P. Tarcher, 1997.

Gray, Bill, *Homeopathy: Science or Myth?,* North Atlantic Books, 2000.

Hershoff, Asa, *Homeopathy for Musculoskeletal Healing,* North Atlantic Books, 1997.

Lansky, Amy L., *Impossible Cure: The Promise of Homeopathy,* R. L. Ranch Pr., 2003.

Lockie, Andrew, and Nicola Geddes, *Complete Guide to Homeopathy: The Principles and Practice of Treatment,* 2nd Ed., Dorling Kindersley Pub., 2002.

Panos, Maesimund, M.D., and Jane Heimlich, *Homeopathic Medicine at Home: Natural Remedies for Everyday Ailments and Minor Injuries,* Jeremy P. Tarcher, 1981.

Ullman, Dana, *Homeopathic Medicine for Children and Infants,* Jeremy P. Tarcher, 1992.

Ullman, Dana, *Homeopathy A-Z,* Hay House Lifestyles, 2002.

Chiropractic

Koch, William H., *Chiropractic: The Superior Alternative,* Bayeux Arts, 1997.

Lenarz, Michael, *The Chiropractic Way: How Chiropractic Care Can Stop Your Pain and Help You Regain Your Health Without Drugs or Surgery,* Bantam, 2003.

McGill, Leonard, *The Chiropractor's Health Book: Simple, Natural Exercises for Relieving Headaches, Tension, and Back Pain,* Three Rivers Press, 1997.

Rondberg, Terry, and Timothy Feuling, *Chiropractic: Compassion and Expectation,* Chiropractic Journal, 1999.

Rondberg, Terry, *Chiropractic First: The Fastest Growing Healthcare Choice Before Drugs or Surgery,* Chiropractic Journal, 1996.

Sportelli, Louis, *Introduction to Chiropractic,* Practicemakers Products Inc., 2000.

Herbal Medicine

Foster, Steven, and Christopher Hobbs, *A Field Guide to Western Medicinal Plants and Herbs,* Houghton Mifflin, 2002.

Gladstar, Rosemary, *Herbal Healing for Women,* Fireside, 1993.

Green, James, *The Male Herbal: Health Care for Men and Boys,* Crossing Press, 1991.

Griggs, Barbara, *Green Pharmacy: The History and Evolution of Western Herbal Medicine,* Healing Arts Press, 1997.

Han, Henry, *Ancient Herbs, Modern Medicine: Improving Your Health by Combining Chinese Herbal Medicine and Western Medicine,* Bantam, 2003.

Hoffman, David, *Complete Illustrated Guide to the Holistic Herbal,* New Ed., Element Books, 2002.

Hoffman, David, *The Herbal Handbook: A User's Guide to Medical Herbalism,* Healing Arts Press, 1998.

Lust, John B., *The Herb Book,* Benedict Lust Publications, 2001.

Molony, David, and Ming Ming Pan Molony, *The American Association of Oriental Medicine's Complete Guide to Chinese Herbal Medicine: How to Treat Illness and Maintain Wellness with Chinese Herbs,* Berkley Publishing Group, 1998.

Tierra, Lesley, *Healing with Chinese Herbs (Crossing Press Healing Series),* Crossing Press, 1997.

Tierra, Lesley, *Herbs of Life: Health and Healing Using Western and Chinese Techniques,* Crossing Press, 1992.

Tilford, Gregory L., *Edible and Medicinal Plants of the West,* Mountain Press Publishing Co., 1997.

Exercise

Bates, Andrea, and Norm Hanson, *Aquatic Exercise Theory*, W.B. Saunders Co., 1996.

Cohen, Ken, *Chi Kung Meditations: Taoist Inner Healing Exercises with Ken Cohen*, Sounds True, 1994 (audio cassette).

Cohen, Ken, *The Way of Qigong: The Art and Science of Chinese Energy Healing*, Wellspring/Ballantine, 1999.

Fenton, Mark, *The 90-Day Fitness Walking Program*, Perigee Books, 1995.

Fenton, Mark, *The Complete Guide to Walking: for Health, Fitness, and Weight Loss*, The Lyons Press, 2001.

Kortge, Carolyn S., *The Spirited Walker: Fitness Walking for Clarity, Balance, and Spiritual Connection*, HarperSanFrancisco, 1998.

Krucoff, Carol, and Mitchell Krucoff, M.D., *Healing Moves: How to Cure, Relieve, and Prevent Common Ailments with Exercise*, Three Rivers Press, 2001.

Malkin, Mort, *Aerobic Walking-The Weight-Loss Exercise: A Complete Program to Reduce Weight, Stress, and Hypertension*, Wiley, 1995.

Man-Ch'ing, Cheng, and Robert W. Smith, *T'ai Chi: The "Supreme Ultimate" Exercise for Health, Sport, and Self-defense*, Tuttle Publishing, 2005.

Menefee, Lynette A., Ph.D., and Daniel R. Somberg, Ph.D., *The Ten Hidden Barriers to Weight Loss and Exercise: Discover Why You've Failed Before and How to Succeed Now*, New Harbinger Publications, 2003.

Neporent, Liz, *Fitness Walking for Dummies*, For Dummies, 1999.

Salmansohn, Karen, *How to Change Your Entire Life By Doing Absolutely Nothing: 10 Do-Nothing Relaxation Exercises to Calm You Down Quickly So You can Speed Forward Faster*, Simon and Schuster, 2003.

Sarley, Ila, and Garrett Sarley, *Walking Yoga: Incorporate Yoga Principles into Dynamic Walking Routines for Physical Health, Mental Peace, and Spiritual Enrichment*, Atria, 2002.

Schlosberg, Suzanne, and Liz Neporent, *Fitness for Dummies,* For Dummies, 2nd Ed., 1999.

Sobel, Dava, and Arthur Klein, *Arthritis, What Exercises Work: Breakthrough Relief for the Rest of Your Life, Even After Drugs and Surgery Have Failed,* St. Martin's Griffin, 1995.

Spilner, Maggie, *Prevention's Complete Book of Walking: Everything You Need to Know to Walk Your Way to Better Health,* Rodale Books, 2000.

Walter, Claire, with Annette Tannander Bank, *The Complete Idiot's Guide to Fitness,* Alpha Books, 2000.

Zhang, Fuxing, *Handbook of T'Ai Chi Ch'Uan Exercises,* Atrium Publishers Group, 1996.

Bodywork

Bentley, Eilean, *Head, Neck & Shoulders Massage: A Step-by-Step Guide,* St. Martin's Press, 2000.

Chow, Kam Thye, *Thai Yoga Massage: A Dynamic Therapy for Physical Well-being and Spiritual Energy,* Healing Arts Press, 2002.

Forem, Jack, and Steve Shimer, *Healing Yourself with Pressure Point Therapy: Simple, Effective Techniques for Massaging Away More than 100 Annoying Ailments,* Prentice Hall, 1999.

Fox, Michael W., *The Healing Touch for Cats: The Proven Massage Program for Cats,* Rev. Ed., Newmarket Press, 2004.

Fox, Michael W., *The Healing Touch for Dogs: The Proven Massage Program for Cats,* Rev. Ed., Newmarket Press, 2004.

Gach, Michael Reed, *Acupressure's Potent Points: a Guide to Self-Care for Common Ailments,* Bantam, 1990.

Gelb, Michael J., *Body Learning: An Introduction to the Alexander Technique,* 2nd Ed., Owl Books, 1996.

Inkeles, Gordon, *Super Massage: Simple Techniques for Instant Relaxation,* 2nd Ed., Arcata Arts, 2001.

Kluck-Ebbin, Michelle, *Hands on Baby Massage,* Running Press Book Publishers, 2004.

Lidell, Lucinda, *The Book of Massage: The Complete Step-by-Step Guide to Eastern and Western Technique,* 2nd Ed., Fireside, 2001.

Menkin, Dan, *Transformation Through Bodywork: Using Touch Therapies for Inner Peace,* Bear & Co., 1996.

Namikoshi, Toru, *The Complete Book of Shiatsu Therapy,* Japan Publications, 1994.

Ohashi, Wataru, *Beyond Shiatsu: Ohashi Bodywork Method,* 2nd Ed., Kodansha America, 2003.

Riggs, Art, *Deep Tissue Massage: A Visual Guide to Techniques,* North Atlantic Books, 2002.

Rosen, Marion, *Rosen Method Bodywork: Accessing the Unconscious Through Touch,* North Atlantic Books, 2003.

Shafarman, Steven, *Awareness Heals: The Feldenkrais Method for Dynamic Health,* Addison Wesley Publishing Co., 1997.

Stillerman, Elaine, *The Encyclopedia of Bodywork: From Acupressure to Zone Therapy,* Checkmark Books, 1997.

Breathwork

Bradley, Dinah, *Self-Help for Hyperventilation Syndrome: Recognizing and Correcting Your Breathing Pattern Disorder,* 3rd Ed., Hunter House, 2001.

Farhi, Donna, *The Breathing Book: Good Health and Vitality Through Essential Breath Work,* Owl Books, 1996.

Fried, Robert L., *Breathe Well, Be Well: A Program to Relieve Stress, Anxiety, Asthma, Hypertension, Migraine, and Other Disorders for Better Health,* Wiley, 1999.

Hale, Teresa, *Breathing Free: The Revolutionary 5-Day Program to Heal Asthma, Emphysema, Bronchitis, and Other Respiratory Ailments,* Three Rivers Press, 2000.

Hendricks, Gay, *Conscious Breathing: Breathwork for Health, Stress Release, and Personal Mastery,* Bantam, 1995.

Lewis, Dennis, *Breathing As a Metaphor for Living: Teachings and Exercises on Complete and Natural Breathing,* Audio Cassette, Sounds True, 1998.

Lewis, Dennis, *The Tao of Natural Breathing: For Health, Well-Being and Inner Growth,* Mountain Wind Publishing, 1996.

Ries, Andrew L., et al., *Shortness of Breath: A Guide to Better Living and Breathing,* 6th Ed., C.V. Mosby, 2000.

Schachter, Neil, *Life and Breath: Preventing, Treating and Reversing Chronic Obstructive Pulmonary Disease.* Broadway, 2003.

Meditation

Allen, Marc, *Stress Reduction and Creative Meditations,* Audio Cassette, New World Library, 1995.

Bodian, Stephan, *Meditation for Dummies,* For Dummies, 1999.

Caponigro, Andy, *The Miracle of the Breath: Mastering Fear, Healing Illness, and Experiencing the Divine,* New World Library, 2005.

Chopra, Deepak, *The Soul of Healing Meditations,* Audio CD, Rasa Music, 2001.

Dalai Lama, *Inner and Outer Peace Through Meditation,* New Ed., Element Books, 2003.

Davich, Victor N., *8 Minute Meditation: Quiet Your Mind, Change Your Life,* Perigee Books, 2004.

Dyer, Wayne W., *Getting in the Gap: Making Conscious Contact with God Through Meditation,* Book with CD, Hay House, 2002.

Kabat-Zinn, Jon, *Wherever You Go, There You Are: Mindfulness Meditation in Everyday Life,* 10th Anniversary Ed., Hyperion, 2005.

Kornfield, Jack, *Meditation for Beginners,* Unabr. Ed., Audio CD, Sounds True, 2001.

MacLean, Kerry Lee, *Peaceful Piggy Meditation,* Albert Whitman and Co., 2004.

MacLean, Kerry Lee, *The Family Meditation Book,* On the Spot! Books, 2004.

Maritza, *Meditation for Beginners,* DVD, Gaiam Americas, 2004.

Yee, Rodney, *Relaxation and Breathing for Meditation,* DVD, Gaiam Americas, 2003.

0-595-35738-5